AF413080

GENERAL AND ABDOMINAL SURGERY

PRACTICES, POTENTIAL COMPLICATIONS AND POSTOPERATIVE MANAGEMENT AND OUTCOMES

SURGERY - PROCEDURES, COMPLICATIONS, AND RESULTS

Additional books in this series can be found on Nova's website under the Series tab.

Additional e-books in this series can be found on Nova's website under the e-book tab.

SURGERY - PROCEDURES, COMPLICATIONS, AND RESULTS

GENERAL AND ABDOMINAL SURGERY

PRACTICES, POTENTIAL COMPLICATIONS AND POSTOPERATIVE MANAGEMENT AND OUTCOMES

KASSANDRA SARAH SLAVOMIR
EDITOR

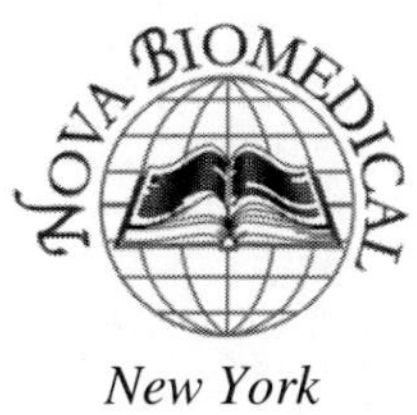

New York

Library of Congress Cataloging-in-Publication Data

ISBN: 978-1-63117-440-7

LCCN: 2014932935

Published by Nova Science Publishers, Inc. † New York

Contents

Preface

Bariatric surgery has become a mainstay in the treatment armamentarium of morbid obesity. Randomized trials have established the efficacy of bariatric surgery towards sustained weight loss, along with significant improvements in related comorbidities, quality of life measures, and all-cause mortality. This compilation discusses the indications and complications of bariatric surgery as well as several other topics that include omentectomy, post surgery atrial fibrillation, blood transfusions, and others.

Chapter 1 - Adipose tissue distribution is an important determinant of obesity-related comorbidities. It is well established that central obesity (intra-abdominal/visceral adipose tissue accumulation) is a risk factor for many adverse metabolic outcomes such as dyslipidemia, hypertension, insulin resistance and type-2-diabetes. Research demonstrates a highly associated link between intra-abdominal (visceral) adipose tissue inflammation and metabolic syndrome, thus the omentum has become an adipose depot of key interest. Indeed, it has been proposed and demonstrated that resection of the omentum, omentectomy, ameliorates metabolic dysregulation, but the results in humans are currently controversial. Despite these controversial results, there is a lack of knowledge about the basic physiological alterations that may occur with removing the omentum in obese or non-obese individuals. It is well established that metabolic improvements following omentum resection are, in part, due to alterations in adipokines (adipocyte hormones that act via autocrine, paracrine, and/or endocrine mechanisms) that were previously dysregulated. Yet, the omentum also contains lymphatic tissue that directly communicates with adipocytes. The role, however, of the lymphatic system/lymph node alterations are underemphasized in omentum resection in obese individuals. In addition to adipose tissue storage the omentum is proposed to function as a peritoneal surveillance for disease and absorber of foreign particulates in peritoneal fluid. For this reason, the inflammatory basis of metabolic syndrome is emerging as interplay between immunological/lymph and adipose tissue. This overview will discuss obesity-induced dysregulation of adipose tissue and lymphatics as well as omentectomy/visceral lipectomy as it pertains to human and rodent research with specific focus on visceral adipose tissue and lymphocyte regulation.

Chapter 2 - Bariatric surgery has become a mainstay in the treatment armamentarium of morbid obesity. Randomized trials have established the efficacy of bariatric surgery towards sustained weight loss, along with significant improvements in related comorbidities, quality of life measures, and all-cause mortality. The most commonly performed and effective procedures include the Laparoscopic Roux-en-Y gastric bypass (LRYGBP), Laparoscopic adjustable gastric banding (LAGB), and Laparoscopic sleeve gastrectomy (LSG). Minimally invasive approaches have become the standard of care as they are associated with smaller incisions, less post-operative pain, fewer respiratory complications, and fewer wound complications.

As with any complex surgical procedure, there are significant complications associated with these operations, including incisional hernias, deep vein thromboses, pulmonary emboli, wound infections, anastomotic leaks, bleeding, and intestinal obstruction. Procedure-specific complications include band slippage, band erosion, internal hernias, dumping syndrome, vitamin deficiencies, marginal ulcers, strictures, and esophageal reflux. Post-operative care in patients with failure of the initial procedure or with complications is challenging and may necessitate revision and reoperation. The author present a brief review of bariatric surgical procedures, discussion of potential complications, and accepted management of these complications.

Chapter 3 - Postoperative atrial fibrillation is a common supraventricular arrhythmia in the context of thoracic cardiac and non-cardiac surgery. In contrast, the incidence of this arrhythmia is very low after non-thoracic non-cardiac surgery. Common risks factor include age, male gender, history of atrial fibrillation, coronary artery disease and atrial enlargement. Inflammation, oxidative stress and surgery-induced release of catecholamines have been implicated in the physiopathology of postoperative atrial fibrillation; hence, several pharmacological interventions have been tried to reduce its incidence. To date, betablockers and amiodarone have shown the most promising benefits in terms of prophylaxis.

Chapter 4 - During the perioperative of any major surgery, there is an intense activation of the sympathetic nervous system, the hypothalamus-pituitary-adrenal axis, and several cellular and soluble components of the inflammatory cascade. All together elements are part so-called stress response. Two characteristics of an exaggerated and uncontrolled stress response are exhaustion and immune suppression. This last, in particular, is relevant in the context of cancer surgery because can lead to growth of any potential postoperative minimal residual disease. To complicate more this matter, anesthetics, opioids and blood transfusions can also contribute to the so-called perioperative immune suppression and cancer growth. Hence, surgeons and anesthesiologist have tried to developed pharmacological and non-pharmacological interventions targeted to avoid the unwanted effects of an exaggerated stress response.

Chapter 5 - The rate of perioperative blood transfusions is still high. They are commonly given to treat perioperative anemia and improve the delivery of oxygen but unfortunately they can also be associated to several adverse reactions. These can range from mild febrile reactions to anaphylactic shock. Less recognized complications associated to the administration of blood products include transfusion-related acute lung injury, graft-versus-host disease, transfusion-related fluid overload and transfusion-related immune suppression. This particular last complication has been the focus of study of several investigators because of the clinical implications on cancer biology, specifically on cancer recurrence. Perturbations in the Th1/Th2 balance and an impaired innate and adaptive immunity are hallmarks of the so-called transfusion related immune suppression. Although, the results from clinical studies evaluating the effects of transfusion-related immune suppression on oncological outcomes are mixed, a meta-analysis in patients with colorectal cancer suggests the association between blood transfusions and cancer recurrence.

Chapter 6 - Gastroesophageal reflux disease (GERD) is a common disease that accounts for the majority of oesophageal pathology. Patients with GERD typically complain of heartburn, regurgitation and/ or dysphagia. Extra-oesophageal symptoms are common and can delay diagnosis and treatment. Several factors may contribute to GERD: Dysfunction of the antireflux barrier, increased oesophageal sensitivity and abnormal oesophageal motility or gastric emptying all play a part in its pathogenesis.

Conservative management is successful in 90% of cases and focuses on lifestyle changes and gastric acid suppression. Proton Pump Inhibitors and histamine- 2- receptor antagonists offer symptomatic relief but their long-term use has been criticized. Other medical treatments (prokinetics, tricyclic anti-depressants) can theoretically improve the symptoms, but the evidence for their use in daily practice, is insufficient.

In specific cases, surgical treatment is indicated. Antireflux surgery aims to restore the gastroesophageal barrier and is an effective way of providing long-term treatment. Nissen fundoplication is the procedure of choice, where the gastric fundus is mobilized and wrapped around the oesophagus (360^0). Different variants of the traditional method (Toupet fundoplication, Belsey Mark IV repair or anterior fundoplication) are recommended in certain cases. Other laparoscopic techniques include the use of magnetic field or electrical stimulation to re-enforce the lower oesophageal sphincter.

Surgical treatment carries the risk of untoward side effects. Besides the common complications of any surgical procedure, fundoplication may be complicated by dysphagia, inability to vomit, increased flactulence, herniation of the repair into the chest and recurrence or persistence of problems.

Chapter 7 - Echinococcosis (hydatid disease) a Zoonosis caused by larval stage of Echinococcus granulosus (also known as Taenia echinococcus). Humans are accidental intermediate hosts,whwreas animals can be both intermediate and definitive hosts. The two main types of hydatid disease are caused by E. granulosus and E. multilocularis. E. granulosus is the most common type of hydatid disease in humans and commonly seen in the Mediterranean, South America, South Africa, Middle east and Australia. Whereas E. multilocularis producing alveolar hydatid disease (alveolar echinococcosis - AE) is limited to certain area of northern hemisphere.

In humans 50-75% of cyst occur in Liver, 25% are located in lungs and less frequently to spleen, kidney, bones, and the brain. Although primary extra-hepatic locations are less common (or even rare in AE), any other organ may be involved. Secondary echinococcosis can develop in the same or other organs. Although less common, AE poses a far more serious problem due to the infiltrative nature of its cysts and its greater ability to metastasise; it has to be regarded as a malignant disease carrying a mortality of up to 90% in untreated cases. Unless otherwise stated in text the authors refer to E. granulosus.

The modern treatment of hydatid cyst of the liver varies from surgical intervention to percutaneous drainage or medical therapy. Surgery is still the treatment of choice and can be performed by the conventional or laparoscopic approach. However, laparoscopic approach leads to an important rate of recurrence of the disease. Percutaneous Aspiration-Injection-Reaspiration Drainage (PAIR) seems to be a better alternative to surgery in selected cases.

In: General and Abdominal Surgery   ISBN: 978-1-63117-440-7
Editor: Kassandra Sarah Slavomir   © 2014 Nova Science Publishers, Inc.

Chapter 1

Omentectomy As a Procedure for the Co-Morbidities of Obesity

***Aaron Magnuson, Andrea Booth
and Michelle Foster**[*]*
Colorado State University, Department of Food Science and Human
Nutrition, Fort Collins, CO, US

Abstract

Adipose tissue distribution is an important determinant of obesity-related comorbidities. It is well established that central obesity (intra-abdominal/visceral adipose tissue accumulation) is a risk factor for many adverse metabolic outcomes such as dyslipidemia, hypertension, insulin resistance and type-2-diabetes. Research demonstrates a highly associated link between intra-abdominal (visceral) adipose tissue inflammation and metabolic syndrome, thus the omentum has become an adipose depot of key interest. Indeed, it has been proposed and demonstrated that resection of the omentum, omentectomy, ameliorates metabolic dysregulation, but the results in humans are currently controversial. Despite these controversial results, there is a lack of knowledge about the basic physiological alterations that may occur with removing the omentum in obese or non-obese individuals. It is well established that metabolic

---

[*] Correspondence: Colorado State University, Department of Food Science and Human Nutrition, Gifford 207, Fort Collins, CO 80523-1571. Email Addresses: Michelle.foster@colostate.edu - Corresponding Author.

improvements following omentum resection are, in part, due to alterations in adipokines (adipocyte hormones that act via autocrine, paracrine, and/or endocrine mechanisms) that were previously dysregulated. Yet, the omentum also contains lymphatic tissue that directly communicates with adipocytes. The role, however, of the lymphatic system/lymph node alterations are underemphasized in omentum resection in obese individuals. In addition to adipose tissue storage the omentum is proposed to function as a peritoneal surveillance for disease and absorber of foreign particulates in peritoneal fluid. For this reason, the inflammatory basis of metabolic syndrome is emerging as interplay between immunological/lymph and adipose tissue. This overview will discuss obesity-induced dysregulation of adipose tissue and lymphatics as well as omentectomy/visceral lipectomy as it pertains to human and rodent research with specific focus on visceral adipose tissue and lymphocyte regulation.

Obesity-Induced Adipose Tissue Dysregulation

Following a harmful stimulus, acute inflammation is the first line of defense in the body's healing process, which consists of a protective immune response to remove damaged cells. It is most commonly characterized by redness, swelling, heat and pain and typically lasts a few days to a week. If the initial inflammatory insult is not resolved, the condition becomes chronic and can often lead to tissue injury. Obesity is characterized as a state of chronic low-grade systemic inflammation occurring as a consequence of intrinsic adipose tissue immune system activation that promotes production and release of proinflammatory cytokines [1]. More specifically, the adipose depot, comprised of adipocytes, stromal vascular preadipocytes and immune cells, is a dynamic tissue that quickly responds to alterations in nutrient intake (i.e., fasting and overfeeding) [2]. Although adipocyte hypertrophy and hyperplasia are typical responses to nutrient overload, accelerated growth or accumulation is recognized as a harmful stimulus and propagates an inflammatory response [3, 4]. This response is perpetuated by dysregulation of adipocytokines [5, 6]. Obesity-induced inflammation initiates locally within the adipose tissue depot, but spreads systemically to other organs in the body (i.e., liver, kidneys, muscle, etc.) [6]. Accordingly, obesity-induced low grade inflammation, in part, is a proposed link to numerous obesity associated co-morbidities such as type-2 diabetes, insulin resistance, dyslipidemia, non-alcoholic fatty liver disease (NAFLD) and cardiovascular disease [7]. The inciting etiology of adipose tissue inflammation and subsequent dysfunction remains to be elucidated. Overall, evidence supports the role of an adipose tissue inflammatory response in the association between obesity and the pathogenesis of chronic metabolic diseases.

Adipose tissue hypoxia, insufficient oxygen supply to expanding and/or proliferating adipocytes, is a proposed inciter of obesity-induced inflammation. During seminal adipocyte expansion, angiogenic factors are increased and subsequent processes in vasculature formation/remodeling are enhanced. The extended vascular network allows uninterrupted delivery of oxygen and nutrients to expanding regions of the adipose depot. Excessive adipose tissue expansion, however, exceeds the availability of angiogenic factors and vasculature development resulting in a reduction of adipose tissue blood flow [8, 9]. Because oxygen diffusion within the adipose depot is limited, decreased blood flow results in hypoxia; this condition occurs in obesity-induce adipocyte growth and proliferation [10]. Insufficient capillary growth/decreased oxygen availability leads to adipocyte dysfunction comprising upregulation of injurious adipokine genes (e.g., TNFα, IL-6, Resistin) and downregulation of beneficial adipokine genes (e.g., adiponectin) and oxidative stress, adipose tissue fibrosis, and eventual cell death/apoptosis [10]. Overall obesity-induced alterations in vasculature function and availability influences adipose tissue homeostasis.

Data supports the hypoxia-induced adipose tissue inflammation postulate, but the direct mechanisms of these responses are not well understood. It has been proposed that adipose tissue hypoxia incites adipocyte dysfunction because it initiates the process of pro-inflammatory cytokine production and immune cell infiltration [11-13]. During obesity-induced inflammation, adipocytes secrete inflammatory cytokines that play a role in maintenance of metabolic dysfunction. Major contributors include monocyte chemoattractant protein 1 (MCP-1), tumor necrosis factor-α (TNFα), and interleukin-6 (IL-6) [8]. MCP-1 serves as the primary recruiter of monocytes from blood vessels surrounding adipose tissue. These monocytes, at maturation are M1 macrophages that produce oxidative metabolites and proinflammatory cytokines in preparation for adipocyte defense [14]. Increased levels of TNFα, as occurs in obesity, are associated with dysregulation of glucose homeostasis and induction of insulin resistance [15, 16]. TNFα also has an inverse relationship to endothelial lipoprotein lipase activity thus it is associated with alterations in lipid metabolism that consequently results in dyslipidemia [17]. Lastly, studies demonstrate TNFα production mediates the production of some adipokines such as leptin and adiponectin [1, 16]. Adipose tissue-derived IL-6 is estimated to make up a third of the total circulating IL-6 in blood, secreted by both adipocytes and macrophages [18]. Unlike TNFα, which acts in an autocrine or paracrine fashion, IL-6 is an endocrine cytokine and plasma concentrations correlate positively with increased lipolysis and insulin resistance [19, 20]. Increased circulating levels of IL-6 are responsible for increased production of C-reactive protein (CRP) by the liver, a strong marker of metabolic risk linked to cardiovascular disease and type-2 diabetes [1].

Dysfunctional lipid metabolism is also an associated co-morbidity of obesity. Lipid dysregulation occurs when requirement for lipid storage exceeds the quantity of adipocyte space, thus perpetuating a milieu favoring inflammation. When lipids exceed adipocyte storage capacity dyslipidemia develops and is characterized by increased levels of triglyceride associated with lipoproteins in the blood [21]. Circulating excess lipid is then transported and ectopically deposited into tissues not designed for lipid storage, such as the liver, kidneys, and/or muscle. In addition, obesity is accompanied by a decrease in insulin signaling which affects multiple tissues including adipocytes by reducing the anti-lipolytic effect of insulin [6]. Consequently, these adipocytes are less effective at storing dietary fatty acids and exacerbate the leak of lipids into the blood. Macrophage infiltration and inflammation-related gene expression, however, occur before the development of insulin resistance in animal models [13, 22-24]. Therefore, adipose tissue lipid dysregulation is not the causal basis of obesity-induced inflammation, but rather, a consequence that contributes to its perpetuation.

Obesity-induced adipocyte dysregulation also leads to disturbances in endocrine regulation of appetite and energy balance. The adipose depot releases biologically active molecules such as adipokines, chemokines, hormone-like factors and numerous other mediators [25]. Adipokines have been demonstrated to affect appetite and satiety, glucose and lipid metabolism, inflammation and immune functions as well as blood pressure [25]. The expression and release of a number of adipokines are increased in the adipose depot with obesity, thus adiposity is connected to dysregulated appetite and metabolism [26]. For example, leptin, a lipostatic signal whose expression directly relates to the proportion of adiposity, is increased with fat accumulation and serves as an anorexigenic signal indicating food intake can be decreased because of positive energy stores [27]. In obesity, leptin receptors in the brain become resistant to the anorexigenic effect of leptin, thus dysregulating appetite and satiety [28]. Other adipokines that play a role in obesity-induced alterations in food intake and regulation of body weight include resistin, visfatin, adipsin and retinal binding protein-4 [29]. In contrast, adiponectin acts as an insulin enhancer and has anti-atherogenic properties. When bound to its receptors, signaling pathways are activated that lead to insulin-sensitization, thus low levels are detrimental to normal glucose function [30]. Circulating adiponectin is decreased in obese individuals and reduced adiponectin has been associated with dyslipidemia and atheroscerosis marked by an increase in CRP, linking the adipose signaling hormone to the inflammatory process [31, 32].

Regional Adipocyte Differences

Traditionally the role of adipose tissue was thought to be limited to storage and insulation. It is now well established that adipose tissue is an immune and endocrine organ that plays a pivotal role in energy homeostasis. The important function of the integrated adipose depot is emphasized by adverse metabolic consequences induced by excessive lipid accumulation. Obesity-related adverse health consequences occur in individuals with predominant upper body adipose distribution [33-37]. This adipose tissue accumulation specifically occurs in the abdominal cavity among organs and is associated with metabolic disorders such as dyslipidemia [38], hypertension [39, 40], insulin resistance and type-2-diabetes [41, 42]. In contrast, increased lower body subcutaneous adipose tissue is associated with a reduced risk of metabolic complications [43] as is upper body subcutaneous fat [44-46]. The mechanisms for this depot distribution and metabolic outcome connection remain to be elucidated, however the proposed mediators commonly attributed to adipocyte dysregulation are excessive accumulation (as previously discussed), location and/or adipose depot intrinsic characteristics.

Intra-abdominal adipose tissue, also known as visceral, includes two distinct depots the mesenteric and omental (Figures 1 and 2). These two central depots are presumed to predispose individuals to adverse health consequences due to their anatomical site that permits venous drainage to the liver via the portal vein; i.e., insulin-sensitive hepatocytes are directly exposed to the metabolites and secretory products released by visceral adipocytes [47-49]. Hence, an increased volume of visceral fat, and subsequent release of fatty acids, glycerol and lactate in addition to numerous adipokines and pro-inflammatory cytokines deposited directly into the portal vein would be expected to have a major influence on these hepatic processes.

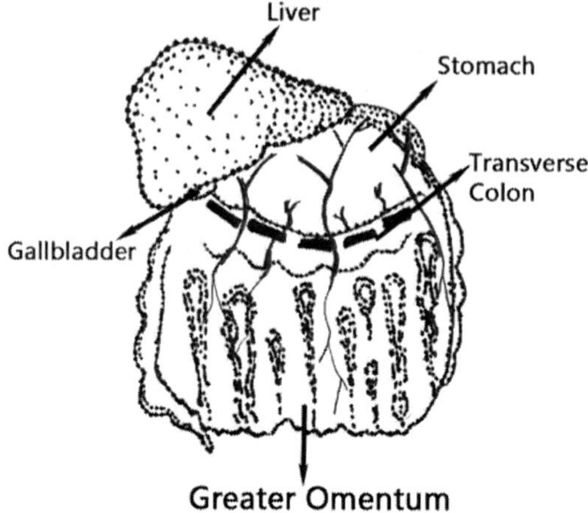

Figure 1.Human Omentum - Omental adipose depot connects the stomach to adjacent organs. The greater omentum, described as "an apron", is suspended from the greater curvature of the stomach and proximal duodenum and extends to the small bowel. The dashed bars represent area of excision for full omentectomy removal.

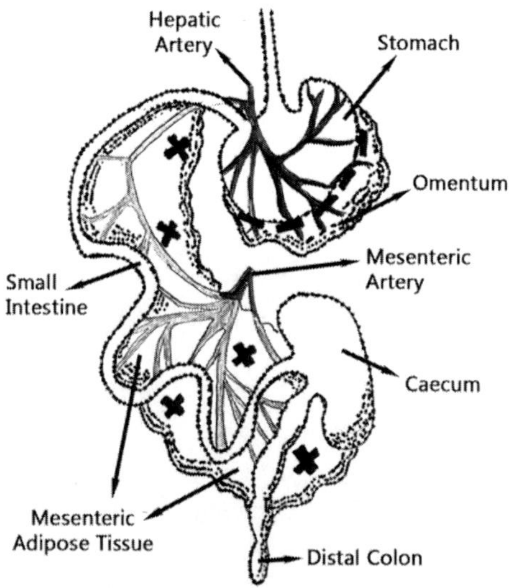

Figure 2. Rodent Visceral Depots (Mesenteric and Omental) – The omentum, suspended from the greater curvature, is relatively small in rodent models and does not connect organs within the abdominal cavity. The mesenteric adipose depot is contained within the mesentery peritoneum that encloses the jejunum and ileum and connects the intestines to the dorsal abdominal wall. The dashed bars represent area of excision for full omentectomy removal, while crosses represent specific sites of mesenteric adipose tissue excision that avoid nerve innervation, vasculature and lymph nodes.

It is well established that lipid influx is an important factor in visceral effluent that influences hepatic processes. Indeed, primary development of insulin resistance is a proposed consequence of enhanced fatty acid release, following excessive visceral adipose tissue accumulation, to the liver via portal circulation. Elevated free fatty acid flux to the liver promotes liver gluconeogenesis [49, 50], reduces enzymes involved in fatty acid oxidation and increases fat storage and synthesis in the liver [51-53] and insulin resistance [53] while decreasing hepatic insulin binding and degradation [54]. These alterations result in systemic hyperinsulinemia [55], attenuation of insulin suppression of hepatic glucose production (i.e., hepatic insulin resistance) [56] and ultimately facilitate hepatic glucose production by providing a continuous source of energy and substrate [56]. Fatty acid-induced dysregulation of insulin-regulated pathways ultimately perpetuates the metabolic effects of obesity by increasing dyslipidemia [57] and ectopic lipid accumulation in the liver [55, 58]. Overall, this suggests that marked central adiposity is one of the main determinants of insulin resistance. This is the basis of Randle's portal/visceral hypothesis which states that increased adiposity, particularly in visceral depots, leads to greater fatty acid flux and inhibition of insulin action in insulin-sensitive tissues [59].

Adipose tissue depots are inherently distinct in structure and metabolic characteristics and these factors create another delineation between the metabolic effects of native adipocytes within the visceral and lower body subcutaneous adipose depots. Adipose tissue depots exhibit differential regulation of triglyceride [60] and fatty acid turnover [61]. These differences are driven by lipolysis rate and adipocyte responsiveness to insulin. When compared to subcutaneous, visceral adipocytes have higher rates of catecholamine-induced lipolysis [62, 63] and express higher numbers of beta adrenergic receptors [64, 65]. Visceral adipocytes are also less responsive to the anti-lipolytic effect of insulin than subcutaneous [66-68] with visceral fat having a lower binding affinity for insulin [69] and reduced insulin receptor substrate (IRS)-1 protein expression [67]. Overall, the lack of sensitivity to insulin can further enhance fatty acid flux to the liver in individuals with visceral obesity.

The differentiation capacity of adipocyte precursor cells varies regionally. Total adipocyte number is regulated via the ratio of apoptosis and development of new cells. As with FA turnover, adipocytes also display a depot-specific susceptibility to apoptosis. More specifically, visceral adipose tissue *in vitro* is more susceptible to tumor necrosis factor (TNF-α), an apoptotic stimulus, than subcutaneous fat [70]. Conversely inhibitors of TNF-α mediated cell death is also expressed at higher levels in visceral than in subcutaneous adipocytes [71]. Visceral adipose tissue also exhibits differences in preadipocyte cell number and differentiation capacity. For example, preadipocytes in confluent cultures from subcutaneous adipose tissue have greater differentiation capacity than those from visceral depots [72]. In sum, visceral fat is characterized by a reduced capacity for differentiation [72] and increased susceptibility to apoptotic stimuli [70] compared with subcutaneous which are factors that could exacerbate an inflammatory environment.

Other intrinsic differences between visceral and subcutaneous adipose tissue include adipokine and cytokine expression, depot configuration and extrinsic factors. More specifically, gene expression [73-75] and release [76, 77] of leptin and adiponectin (adipokines previously discussed) is higher in subcutaneous adipose tissue than visceral. In opposition, the visceral depot exhibits an enhanced inflammatory profile with increased cytokine expression, specifically IL-6, IL-8, PAI-1, MCP-1 and Visfatin, compared with subcutaneous (for a review see ref [78]). Differences in depot characteristics also extend to adipocyte architecture, connective tissue, and additional cells such as macrophages and immune and stromovascular cells within the depot [79, 80]. Extrinsic factors including, but not limited to, vasculature/angiogenic capacity, innervation/lipolysis drive and lymphatic/immune stimulation are once again higher in the visceral depot, which is likely due to intestinal/gut proximity [81, 82].

Omentectomy As a Treatment for Obesity

Visceral adipose tissue consists of two depots, the mesenteric and the omental. The mesenteric adipose depot is contained within the mesentery peritoneum that encloses the jejunum and ileum and connects the intestines to the dorsal abdominal wall. The omentum peritoneum (Figure 1) that encases the omental adipose depot connects the stomach to adjacent organs. Peritoneal extensions of this region are divided into greater and lesser portions. The lesser peritoneal connects the lesser curvature of the stomach and proximal duodenum with the liver, whereas the greater peritoneal is suspended from the greater curvature of the stomach and proximal duodenum and extends to the small bowel. Unlike the lesser omentum and mesenteric peritoneal, the greater omentum, often described as "an apron", is mobile and freely moves around the peritoneal cavity. This abdominal sheet is composed primarily of adipose tissue, but also contains gastroepiploic and lymphatic vessels.

As previously discussed visceral adipose tissue accumulation, mesenteric and omental, is highly associated with the co-morbidities of obesity unlike lower body subcutaneous adipose deposition which is suggested to be "protective". Hence visceral removal in obese subjects could attenuate obesity co-morbidities such as insulin resistance, inflammation and glucose intolerance. The mesenteric depot in humans, however, cannot be surgically removed without risk of complications [83]. In contrast, the omentum because of its anatomical location can be removed with ease. The omentum, previously thought to perform no important functions, plays a role in energy regulation by influencing glucose and fatty acid metabolism.

Omentectomy (i.e., removal of all or part of the greater omentum and its constituent fat) (Figure 1) has unclear physiological implications in humans. Whereas some human studies demonstrate omental fat removal improves insulin action [83, 84] in obese patients, others observe no alterations [85, 86]. The conflicting results are likely due to inherent experimental limitations and individual variation between humans. For example, the omentectomy procedure is rarely individually executed and is often associated with gastric bypass or banding or intestine removal [83-86]. Thus the accelerated weight loss due to the additional procedures could mask the effects of omental fat removal. Other factors that may contribute to these contradictions include variations in pre- and post-operative BMI or body mass, amount of adipose tissue removed, age, sex, and duration of study.

In rodents, selective reduction in intra-abdominal adipose tissue improves metabolic profile. Specifically, intra-abdominal lipectomy (adipose tissue removal) reverses insulin resistance and glucose intolerance in obese, aged and young rodents [87-92]. Most rodent studies, however, are an inadequate representation of human omentectomy. First, in rodent models, the removed intra-abdominal adipose depot is attached to the reproductive organs rather than to portal drainage to the liver [93] and no human equivalent. Second, the rodent omentum is not equivalent in size to the human omentum; it is minuscule, often negligible in lean animals. Still, visceral lipectomy in rodents is a useful tool to investigate whether visceral obesity is a consequence or a contributing factor of the co-morbidities of obesity. Despite the omental difference, human omentectomy can be mimicked in the rodent by excising the whole omentum and portions of the mesenteric depot (Figure 2) [94]. In the latter, care must be taken to avoid removal of vasculature, lymph drainage or nerves that innervate the intestine. Visceral adipose tissue (*i.e* omental and mesenteric) removal in rodents improves glucose tolerance and reduces liver triglyceride storage [94]. Deleterious effects of an expanding visceral depot are proposed to be a result of the visceral effluent, such as free fatty acids and adipocytokines, which affect insulin-sensitive hepatocytes [47-49]. Despite the location of intra-abdominal adipose tissue removal, these studies demonstrate that free fatty acids and adipo/cytokines play prominent roles in fat removal-induced improvements in insulin signaling and glucose homeostasis [87-92]. The long-term impact, however, of visceral adipose tissue removal in rodents and humans is currently unknown.

Although omentectomy is a procedure of interest for obesity treatment it is most commonly utilized in many cancer-staging procedures (pathological evaluation to determine the severity of cancer). These include, but are not limited to, primary peritoneal, ovarian, fallopian tube and gastric cancers [95-97]. Despite the vast use of omentectomy in abdominal cancer procedures or its investigational use as a potential treatment for obesity the long-term post-operative consequences remain unknown. Although necessity may outweigh the potential negative consequences of greater omentum removal in cancer patients it is essential to understand effects of this surgery in relation to the co-morbidities of obesity.

The Omentum and Immunity

Visceral adipose tissue accumulation is highly associated with greater risk for metabolic and cardiovascular disease, thus its removal may reverse these pathological conditions. Omentectomy, however, removes more than just visceral adipocytes. The omentum, which is bathed in the peritoneal fluid, is proposed to be a "peritoneal surveillance system" which serves to shield and limit abnormalities in the intra-abdominal cavity such as infectious and inflammatory processes and neoplastic intraperitneal dispersion. This protective role, however, is often underemphasized in obesity treatment omentectomy where the outcome measurements focus primarily on glucose tolerance, insulin sensitivity, circulating lipids, weight/BMI and adipocytokines. There has been little consideration to the long-term effects of omentum removal on immunity homeostasis.

The omentum is a physiologically dynamic tissue with therapeutic potential. It predominantly consists of adipose tissue, but also contains blood vessels and lymphatic/cellular tissues that are an integral part of the immune system defending the peritoneal cavity. The omental lymphatic system helps to clean and maintain proper function of organs in the abdominal cavity via absorbing edema fluids and removing metabolic waste and toxic substances (i.e., bacteria or other contaminants that enter the cavity from the small intestine and colon) [98]. Within the fatty omenta are capsule encased lymph nodes and numerous secondary lymphoid opaque structures called milky spots [99]. The lymph node is split into three compartments; the cortex, paracortex, and medulla. Housed within these three compartments are lymphocytes, B and T cells, antigen presenting cells and macrophages (Figure 3) [100]. Here the naive B and T cells become mature and undergo clonal expansion after interacting with antigen presenting cells and subsequently defend against infection and/or neoplastic intraperitneal dispersion [100]. Mature B-lymphocytes primary action is the release of antibodies (IgG, IgM, IgA, IgE, and IgD) that bind foreign antigens; each B cell produces a single programmed recognition reaction out of hundreds of millions of possibilities [40]. T-cells, unlike B cells, do not recognize full antigens, but rather fragments of antigens present on the surface of damaged cells (i.e., those infected by virus or cancerous cells). T-cells also differ from B-cells by their ability to enter cells infected or infiltrated by an infectious agent [40]. The T-cell population can be further subdivided relative to primary function. For example, there are those that direct immune response such as the T-lymphocytes and T-helper cells and others that directly attack infected or mutated cells like cytotoxic T-lymphocytes and natural killer cells. A host of other cells are also involved in the generalized immune response such as granulocytes and mast cells [40]. Immune cells contained within lymph nodes are distributed throughout the body via lymphatic veinules, a bidirectional transport network carrying lymph fluid out and inflammatory mediators, antigenic materials and antigen presenting cells in [100].

As previously mentioned the omentum also contains secondary lymphoid structures called milky spots [99, 101]. These spots primarily consist of macrophages (immune cells that ingest or phagocytize antigenic material), but also include T-lymphocytes, stromal and mast cells and a site-specific subset of B lymphocytes [102, 103]. Hence the populations of cells within the milky spots differ from those that are found in the lymph nodes. Milky spots, regarded as a main source of peritoneal macrophages [104], primary function is to clear particles, bacteria and tumor cells from the peritoneal cavity [105-107]. Macrophages within milky spots, yet to encounter foreign antigenic material, remain quiescent until an antigen is introduced. Once activated these macrophages present the antigens to naïve lymphocytes to initiate maturation. Accordingly the lymph node is the site of maturation for lymphocytes that interact with antigen presenting cells, thus macrophages present antigens that can then be recognized by lymphocytes in the immune response [65, 66]. Once these interactions occur, the lymphocytes travel out of the lymph node and circulate throughout the body and peritoneal cavity [99]. In general milky spots are a collection area for antigens that allows fast exchange of quarantined foreign material and initiation of immune response. They differ from lymph nodes in development, morphology and immunological properties [99, 108] and are specifically suited for migration of leukocytes and rapid movement of fluids.

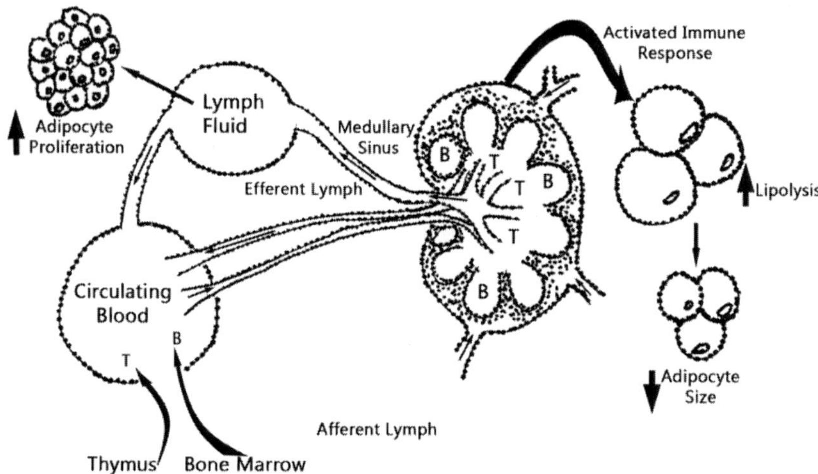

Figure 3. Adipose Tissue-Lymph Node Crosstalk – T and B-lymphocytes produced in the thymus and bone marrow enter peripheral lymph tissue via blood circulation. Once in the lymph node naive B-lymphocytes reside in the primary follicles of the cortical lymphoid follicles, whereas T cells reside mainly in the paracortical area. In the presence of an activated immune response energy is derived from free fatty acids released from adipocytes following an increase in adipose lipolysis. This ultimately results in a decrease in perinodal adipocyte cell size. Lymph fluid has been demonstrated to increase adipocyte proliferation.

Adipose Tissue - Lymph Node Crosstalk

As previously discussed virtually all mammalian lymphatic vessels and nodes are in close spatial association with adipose tissue [109]. Adipocytes in close proximity to lymph nodes, termed "perinodal", are found roughly within a 2mm radius [110]. Adipocytes further out are designated "middle", 5-10mm from node, or "outside" at the distance of 10mm or greater. Perinodal adipocytes have been demonstrated to be a reservoir of energy for lymphatic vessels and structures needed to deploy an immune response [111]. Both lymphocytes and tissue-derived dendritic cells utilize this energy from fatty acid metabolism (Figure 3). Dendritic cells that increase in number following chronic immune stimulation/inflammation [112] are a specific set of antigen presenting cells that function to activate specific immune responses involved with T-cells [113]. Studies demonstrate that chronic inflammation of lymph nodes, immune stimulation, increases lipolysis in perinodal adipocytes and subsequently decreases adipocyte cell size [109]. This local interaction with adipocyte liberated lipids, free fatty acids, subsequently nourish and/or regulate lymphocytes. In contrast, immune stimulation has also been demonstrated to increase perinodal adipogenic activity. Indeed, chronic inflammation of lymph nodes in rats increases the number of adipocytes surrounding the nodes [114]. Lymph fluid can also promote differentiation of preadipocytes [115]. For example, abnormal lymph leakage due to disruption in lymphatic vascular integrity promotes ectopic growth of adipose tissue due to increased lipid storage in adipocytes and increased differentiation of preadipocytes [116]. Another study observed ectopic adipose growth in edematous regions of individuals with chronic lymphedema [117]. Overall, adipocytes that surround lymph nodes are actively involved in the transient immune response, explaining the spatial relationship of adipose tissue to lymph vessels.

The Healing Omentum

The role of the omentum in peritoneal defense is, in part, due to immunity, but also a supportive role in repairing tissue damage. The omentum has the ability to adhere to sites of inflammation on adjacent organs and subsequently destroy pathogens and repair damaged tissue [98, 102]. Indeed, the omentum is a source of growth factors, neurotransmitters, neurotrophic factors and inflammatory mediators that help to promote tissue regeneration [98, 118]. The healing qualities are due to stem cell production within this tissue permitting subsequent tissue regeneration of surrounding organs after damage occurs [118]. Based on its inherent defense mechanisms and its angiogenic ability to help seal off and repair damaged or infected tissues the omentum has potent healing properties and for this reason has been used by surgeons for some time. Clinically, cells from the omentum have been used for healing and tissue regeneration in procedures such as, but not limited to, gastrointestinal [119], neuro- [120], cardiothoracic [121], gynecological [122] and urological

[123] surgeries. Omental fixation or wrapping to cover or surround tissue is an effective method of minimizing post-operative complications, surgical morbidity or infection while enhancing vascularization and tissue restoration. Omentum interposition has wide therapeutic application in many branches of surgery.

Implications of Omentum Removal in Obesity

The omentum is a versatile organ demonstrated to play a role in peritoneal defense by way of antigen removal and tissue repair. The importance of this role, however, is underemphasized in obesity-treatment surgeries (i.e., bariatric surgery) with concomitant omentum removal, instead the primary focus is placed on adipocyte dysregulation. Although adipose tissue hypoxia is proposed to incite obesity co-morbidities, growing evidence suggest the small intestine, the first interface between the body and diet, contributes greatly to the development of metabolic disease [124]. Indeed, the contribution of gut microbiota, microorganisms in the digestive tract, is gaining increased recognition. Gut microbiota component lipopolysaccharide (LPS), the main constituent of the outer membrane of Gram-negative bacteria, causes immune system activation. LPS, an endotoxin, is a major inducer of the inflammatory response and is increased in blood circulation following chronic fat ingestion because diets high in fat cause increased gastrointestinal permeability (increased gut leakage) [125]. In the peritoneal cavity endotoxaemia triggers an innate response that causes the release of proinflammatory cytokines that subsequently interferes with whole body glucose and lipid metabolism. Although lymph nodes are the nexus of the gastrointestinal tract and adipose tissue, its role is often underemphasized despite being fundamental.

As previously discussed, central obesity is highly associated with metabolic dysregulation. Proposed fundamental obesity-induced triggers or aggravators include adipose depot increases in deleterious adipokines, cytokines, free fatty acid leakage and inflammation. Recent studies also demonstrate peritoneal lymphatics play a role in the development of obesity-associated co-morbidities. For example, diet-induced and genetic obesity increases lymph node associated T-lymphocytes [126, 127], mast cells (immune cell with granules that contain histamine and heparin) and immune cell apoptosis [128]. Some, however, demonstrate obesity induces decreases in

T-lymphocytes while exacerbating immune responses by enhancing T-cell activation [129]. Increased lymph node mast cell density may further incite exacerbation by activating lymph nodes [130] and facilitating the recruitment of T-lymphocytes [131]. These chronic changes ultimately lead to apoptosis of crucial cells that play a role in immune homeostasis. Indeed, lymphoid cellularity of diet-induced obese mice declines as mesenteric adipose tissue accumulates resulting in atrophy of lymph node structures [132]. Alterations of lymphatic tissue and associated cells are proposed to be initiated by the surrounding microenvironment that is dictated by adjacent adipocytes and peritoneal fluid.

In obese humans, omentectomy with and perhaps without bariatric surgery, may reverse metabolic co-morbidities in a multifaceted way. First, omentum removal decreases the amount of hypoxic visceral adipose tissue. Consequently, deleterious factors released from impaired adipocytes (e.g., adipocytokines and free fatty acids) within the omentum depot are no longer part of the effluent to the liver. Second, omentectomy also includes removal of dysregulated lymphatics, milky spots and lymph nodes, responsible for exacerbating the cycle of immune injury. Therefore, the removal of this one visceral depot alone may be adequate in reversing the co-morbidities of obesity, but success of this procedure may be dependent upon appropriate food intake and maintenance of a healthy weight. Specifically, if the omentum is dysregulated it is likely the other visceral depot, mesenteric, is too. Hence, if the omental depot is removed, but energy excess and need for adipose tissue storage continues, energy surplus will likely be shunted to the mesenteric depot. The mesenteric depot is susceptible to obesity-induced alterations and like the omentum contains lymph nodes that can become impaired [133], however the progression of these events in human mesenteric is unknown. Yet, it is plausible that omentectomy without subsequent weight loss or reduction in calories would not attenuate the co-morbidities of obesity in the long-term because the mesenteric depot remains intact. The beneficial effects of omentectomy would be greater if combined with gastric bypass, assuring weight loss occurs and is maintained. Current human research is unclear about omentectomy as a procedure for the co-morbidities of obesity. Follow-up studies should investigate effects of adiposity distribution, specifically discerning the quantity of omental and mesenteric adipose tissue, and systematically observe mesenteric alterations (e.g., quantitiy) and circulating adipocytokine and endotoxin concentration following omental depot removal.

References

[1]   B. E. Wisse, The inflammatory syndrome: the role of adipose tissue cytokines in metabolic disorders linked to obesity. *Journal of the American Society of Nephrology : JASN* 15, 2792-2800 (2004); published online EpubNov (10.1097/01.ASN.0000141966.69934.21).

[2]   N. Halberg, I. Wernstedt-Asterholm, P. E. Scherer, The adipocyte as an endocrine cell. *Endocrinology and metabolism clinics of North America* 37, 753-768, x-xi (2008); published online EpubSep (10.1016 /j.ecl.2008.07.002).

[3]   J. Jo, O. Gavrilova, S. Pack, W. Jou, S. Mullen, A. E. Sumner, S. W. Cushman, V. Periwal, Hypertrophy and/or Hyperplasia: Dynamics of Adipose Tissue Growth. *PLoS computational biology* 5, e1000324 (2009); published online EpubMar (10.1371/journal.pcbi.1000324).

[4]   H. E. Bays, J. M. Gonzalez-Campoy, G. A. Bray, A. E. Kitabchi, D. A. Bergman, A. B. Schorr, H. W. Rodbard, R. R. Henry, Pathogenic potential of adipose tissue and metabolic consequences of adipocyte hypertrophy and increased visceral adiposity. *Expert review of cardiovascular therapy* 6, 343-368 (2008); published online EpubMar (10.1586/14779072.6.3.343).

[5]   S. P. Weisberg, D. McCann, M. Desai, M. Rosenbaum, R. L. Leibel, A. W. Ferrante, Jr., Obesity is associated with macrophage accumulation in adipose tissue. *J Clin Invest* 112, 1796-1808 (2003); published online EpubDec (10.1172/JCI19246).

[6]   G. H. Goossens, The role of adipose tissue dysfunction in the pathogenesis of obesity-related insulin resistance. *Physiol Behav* 94, 206-218 (2008); published online EpubMay 23 (10.1016 /j.physbeh.2007.10.010).

[7]   G. S. Hotamisligil, Inflammation and metabolic disorders. *Nature* 444, 860-867 (2006); published online EpubDec 14 (10.1038/nature05485).

[8]   P. Trayhurn, B. Wang, I. S. Wood, Hypoxia and the endocrine and signalling role of white adipose tissue. *Archives of physiology and biochemistry* 114, 267-276 (2008); published online EpubOct (10.1080/13813450802306602).

[9]   J. Ye, Emerging role of adipose tissue hypoxia in obesity and insulin resistance. *Int J Obes (Lond)* 33, 54-66 (2009); published online EpubJan (10.1038/ijo.2008.229).

[10] P. Trayhurn, Hypoxia and adipose tissue function and dysfunction in obesity. *Physiol Rev* 93, 1-21 (2013); published online EpubJan (10.1152/physrev.00017.2012).

[11] R. W. O'Rourke, A. E. White, M. D. Metcalf, A. S. Olivas, P. Mitra, W. G. Larison, E. C. Cheang, O. Varlamov, C. L. Corless, C. T. Roberts, Jr., D. L. Marks, Hypoxia-induced inflammatory cytokine secretion in human adipose tissue stromovascular cells. *Diabetologia* 54, 1480-1490 (2011); published online EpubJun (10.1007/s00125-011-2103-y).

[12] J. Ye, Z. Gao, J. Yin, Q. He, Hypoxia is a potential risk factor for chronic inflammation and adiponectin reduction in adipose tissue of ob/ob and dietary obese mice. *American journal of physiology. Endocrinology and metabolism* 293, E1118-1128 (2007); published online EpubOct (10.1152/ajpendo.00435.2007).

[13] P. Trayhurn, I. S. Wood, Adipokines: inflammation and the pleiotropic role of white adipose tissue. *Br J Nutr* 92, 347-355 (2004); published online EpubSep.

[14] A. H. Ding, C. F. Nathan, D. J. Stuehr, Release of reactive nitrogen intermediates and reactive oxygen intermediates from mouse peritoneal macrophages. Comparison of activating cytokines and evidence for independent production. *Journal of immunology* 141, 2407-2412 (1988); published online EpubOct 1.

[15] G. S. Hotamisligil, P. Arner, J. F. Caro, R. L. Atkinson, B. M. Spiegelman, Increased adipose tissue expression of tumor necrosis factor-alpha in human obesity and insulin resistance. *J Clin Invest* 95, 2409-2415 (1995); published online EpubMay (10.1172/JCI117936).

[16] J. K. Sethi, G. S. Hotamisligil, The role of TNF alpha in adipocyte metabolism. *Seminars in cell & developmental biology* 10, 19-29 (1999); published online EpubFeb (10.1006/scdb.1998.0273).

[17] P. A. Kern, M. Saghizadeh, J. M. Ong, R. J. Bosch, R. Deem, R. B. Simsolo, The expression of tumor necrosis factor in human adipose tissue. Regulation by obesity, weight loss, and relationship to lipoprotein lipase. *J Clin Invest* 95, 2111-2119 (1995); published online EpubMay (10.1172/JCI117899).

[18] K. Eder, N. Baffy, A. Falus, A. K. Fulop, The major inflammatory mediator interleukin-6 and obesity. *Inflammation research : official journal of the European Histamine Research Society ... [et al.]* 58, 727-736 (2009); published online EpubNov (10.1007/s00011-009-0060-4).

[19] G. van Hall, A. Steensberg, M. Sacchetti, C. Fischer, C. Keller, P. Schjerling, N. Hiscock, K. Moller, B. Saltin, M. A. Febbraio, B. K.

Pedersen, Interleukin-6 stimulates lipolysis and fat oxidation in humans. *J Clin Endocrinol Metab* 88, 3005-3010 (2003); published online EpubJul.

[20] P. A. Kern, S. Ranganathan, C. Li, L. Wood, G. Ranganathan, Adipose tissue tumor necrosis factor and interleukin-6 expression in human obesity and insulin resistance. *American journal of physiology. Endocrinology and metabolism* 280, E745-751 (2001); published online EpubMay.

[21] J. O. Ebbert, M. D. Jensen, Fat depots, free fatty acids, and dyslipidemia. *Nutrients* 5, 498-508 (2013); published online EpubFeb (10.3390 /nu5020498).

[22] J. S. Yudkin, C. D. Stehouwer, J. J. Emeis, S. W. Coppack, C-reactive protein in healthy subjects: associations with obesity, insulin resistance, and endothelial dysfunction: a potential role for cytokines originating from adipose tissue? *Arteriosclerosis, thrombosis, and vascular biology* 19, 972-978 (1999); published online EpubApr.

[23] A. Festa, R. D'Agostino, Jr., K. Williams, A. J. Karter, E. J. Mayer-Davis, R. P. Tracy, S. M. Haffner, The relation of body fat mass and distribution to markers of chronic inflammation. *Int J Obes Relat Metab Disord* 25, 1407-1415 (2001); published online EpubOct (10.1038/sj.ijo.0801792).

[24] G. S. Hotamisligil, Inflammatory pathways and insulin action. *Int J Obes Relat Metab Disord* 27 Suppl 3, S53-55 (2003); published online EpubDec (10.1038/sj.ijo.0802502).

[25] S. E. Wozniak, L. L. Gee, M. S. Wachtel, E. E. Frezza, Adipose tissue: the new endocrine organ? A review article. *Digestive diseases and sciences* 54, 1847-1856 (2009); published online EpubSep (10.1007/s10620-008-0585-3).

[26] J. P. Bastard, M. Maachi, C. Lagathu, M. J. Kim, M. Caron, H. Vidal, J. Capeau, B. Feve, Recent advances in the relationship between obesity, inflammation, and insulin resistance. *European cytokine network* 17, 4-12 (2006); published online EpubMar.

[27] M. Maffei, J. Halaas, E. Ravussin, R. E. Pratley, G. H. Lee, Y. Zhang, H. Fei, S. Kim, R. Lallone, S. Ranganathan, et al., Leptin levels in human and rodent: measurement of plasma leptin and ob RNA in obese and weight-reduced subjects. *Nat Med* 1, 1155-1161 (1995); published online EpubNov.

[28] H. Munzberg, M. Bjornholm, S. H. Bates, M. G. Myers, Jr., Leptin receptor action and mechanisms of leptin resistance. *Cellular and*

molecular life sciences : CMLS 62, 642-652 (2005); published online EpubMar (10.1007/s00018-004-4432-1).

[29] E. E. Kershaw, J. S. Flier, Adipose tissue as an endocrine organ. *J Clin Endocrinol Metab* 89, 2548-2556 (2004); published online EpubJun (10.1210/jc.2004-0395).

[30] A. S. Lihn, S. B. Pedersen, B. Richelsen, Adiponectin: action, regulation and association to insulin sensitivity. *Obesity reviews : an official journal of the International Association for the Study of Obesity* 6, 13-21 (2005); published online EpubFeb (10.1111/j.1467-789X.2005.00159.x).

[31] G. Fantuzzi, Adiponectin and inflammation: consensus and controversy. *The Journal of allergy and clinical immunology* 121, 326-330 (2008); published online EpubFeb (10.1016/j.jaci.2007.10.018).

[32] N. Ouchi, K. Walsh, A novel role for adiponectin in the regulation of inflammation. *Arteriosclerosis, thrombosis, and vascular biology* 28, 1219-1221 (2008); published online EpubJul (10.1161 /ATVBAHA.108.165068).

[33] P. Bjorntorp, Metabolic implications of body fat distribution. *Diabetes Care* 14, 1132-1143 (1991); published online EpubDec.

[34] A. H. Kissebah, G. R. Krakower, Regional adiposity and morbidity. *Physiol Rev* 74, 761-811 (1994); published online EpubOct.

[35] J. Vague, The degree of masculine differentiation of obesities: a factor determining predisposition to diabetes, atherosclerosis, gout, and uric calculous disease. *Am J Clin Nutr* 4, 20-34 (1956); published online EpubJan-Feb.

[36] P. Bjorntorp, "Portal" adipose tissue as a generator of risk factors for cardiovascular disease and diabetes. *Arteriosclerosis* 10, 493-496 (1990); published online EpubJul-Aug.

[37] M. T. Foster, M. J. Pagliassotti, Metabolic alterations following visceral fat removal and expansion: Beyond anatomic location. *Adipocyte* 1, 192-199 (2012); published online EpubOct 1 (10.4161/adip.21756).

[38] A. H. Kissebah, S. Alfarsi, P. W. Adams, V. Wynn, Role of insulin resistance in adipose tissue and liver in the pathogenesis of endogenous hypertriglyceridaemia in man. *Diabetologia* 12, 563-571 (1976); published online EpubDec.

[39] P. A. Cassano, M. R. Segal, P. S. Vokonas, S. T. Weiss, Body fat distribution, blood pressure, and hypertension. A prospective cohort study of men in the normative aging study. *Ann Epidemiol* 1, 33-48 (1990); published online EpubOct.

[40] J. C. Seidell, M. Cigolini, J. P. Deslypere, J. Charzewska, B. M. Ellsinger, A. Cruz, Body fat distribution in relation to serum lipids and blood pressure in 38-year-old European men: the European fat distribution study. *Atherosclerosis* 86, 251-260 (1991); published online EpubFeb.

[41] V. J. Carey, E. E. Walters, G. A. Colditz, C. G. Solomon, W. C. Willett, B. A. Rosner, F. E. Speizer, J. E. Manson, Body fat distribution and risk of non-insulin-dependent diabetes mellitus in women. The Nurses' Health Study. *Am J Epidemiol* 145, 614-619 (1997); published online EpubApr 1.

[42] J. M. Chan, E. B. Rimm, G. A. Colditz, M. J. Stampfer, W. C. Willett, Obesity, fat distribution, and weight gain as risk factors for clinical diabetes in men. *Diabetes Care* 17, 961-969 (1994); published online EpubSep.

[43] M. B. Snijder, J. M. Dekker, M. Visser, L. M. Bouter, C. D. Stehouwer, J. S. Yudkin, R. J. Heine, G. Nijpels, J. C. Seidell, Trunk fat and leg fat have independent and opposite associations with fasting and postload glucose levels: the Hoorn study. *Diabetes Care* 27, 372-377 (2004); published online EpubFeb.

[44] W. T. Cefalu, Z. Q. Wang, S. Werbel, A. Bell-Farrow, J. R. Crouse, 3rd, W. H. Hinson, J. G. Terry, R. Anderson, Contribution of visceral fat mass to the insulin resistance of aging. *Metabolism* 44, 954-959 (1995); published online EpubJul.

[45] J. C. Seidell, P. Bjorntorp, L. Sjostrom, H. Kvist, R. Sannerstedt, Visceral fat accumulation in men is positively associated with insulin, glucose, and C-peptide levels, but negatively with testosterone levels. *Metabolism* 39, 897-901 (1990); published online EpubSep.

[46] J. L. Kuk, P. T. Katzmarzyk, M. Z. Nichaman, T. S. Church, S. N. Blair, R. Ross, Visceral fat is an independent predictor of all-cause mortality in men. *Obesity (Silver Spring)* 14, 336-341 (2006); published online EpubFeb.

[47] G. S. Hotamisligil, P. Peraldi, A. Budavari, R. Ellis, M. F. White, B. M. Spiegelman, IRS-1-mediated inhibition of insulin receptor tyrosine kinase activity in TNF-alpha- and obesity-induced insulin resistance. *Science* 271, 665-668 (1996); published online EpubFeb 2.

[48] R. N. Bergman, Non-esterified fatty acids and the liver: why is insulin secreted into the portal vein? *Diabetologia* 43, 946-952 (2000); published online EpubJul.

[49] J. R. Williamson, R. A. Kreisberg, P. W. Felts, Mechanism for the stimulation of gluconeogenesis by fatty acids in perfused rat liver. *Proc Natl Acad Sci U S A* 56, 247-254 (1966); published online EpubJul (

[50] J. R. Williamson, Mechanism for the stimulation in vivo of hepatic gluconeogenesis by glucagon. *Biochem J* 101, 11C-14C (1966); published online EpubOct.

[51] S. D. Clarke, Polyunsaturated fatty acid regulation of gene transcription: a mechanism to improve energy balance and insulin resistance. *Br J Nutr* 83 Suppl 1, S59-66 (2000); published online EpubMar.

[52] J. Xu, M. T. Nakamura, H. P. Cho, S. D. Clarke, Sterol regulatory element binding protein-1 expression is suppressed by dietary polyunsaturated fatty acids. A mechanism for the coordinate suppression of lipogenic genes by polyunsaturated fats. *J Biol Chem* 274, 23577-23583 (1999); published online EpubAug 13.

[53] N. D. Oakes, G. J. Cooney, S. Camilleri, D. J. Chisholm, E. W. Kraegen, Mechanisms of liver and muscle insulin resistance induced by chronic high-fat feeding. *Diabetes* 46, 1768-1774 (1997); published online EpubNov.

[54] J. Svedberg, P. Bjorntorp, U. Smith, P. Lonnroth, Free-fatty acid inhibition of insulin binding, degradation, and action in isolated rat hepatocytes. *Diabetes* 39, 570-574 (1990); published online EpubMay.

[55] R. L. Dobbins, L. S. Szczepaniak, B. Bentley, V. Esser, J. Myhill, J. D. McGarry, Prolonged inhibition of muscle carnitine palmitoyltransferase-1 promotes intramyocellular lipid accumulation and insulin resistance in rats. *Diabetes* 50, 123-130 (2001); published online EpubJan.

[56] G. Boden, Role of fatty acids in the pathogenesis of insulin resistance and NIDDM. *Diabetes* 46, 3-10 (1997); published online EpubJan.

[57] P. J. Voshol, P. C. Rensen, K. W. van Dijk, J. A. Romijn, L. M. Havekes, Effect of plasma triglyceride metabolism on lipid storage in adipose tissue: Studies using genetically engineered mouse models. *Biochim Biophys Acta*, (2009); published online EpubJan 8.

[58] L. Heilbronn, S. R. Smith, E. Ravussin, Failure of fat cell proliferation, mitochondrial function and fat oxidation results in ectopic fat storage, insulin resistance and type II diabetes mellitus. *Int J Obes Relat Metab Disord* 28 Suppl 4, S12-21 (2004); published online EpubDec.

[59] P. J. Randle, P. B. Garland, C. N. Hales, E. A. Newsholme, The glucose fatty-acid cycle. Its role in insulin sensitivity and the metabolic disturbances of diabetes mellitus. *Lancet* 1, 785-789 (1963); published online EpubApr 13.

[60] M. D. Jensen, Health consequences of fat distribution. *Horm Res* 48 Suppl 5, 88-92 (1997).

[61] J. Ostman, P. Arner, P. Engfeldt, L. Kager, Regional differences in the control of lipolysis in human adipose tissue. *Metabolism* 28, 1198-1205 (1979); published online EpubDec.

[62] M. Rebuffe-Scrive, B. Andersson, L. Olbe, P. Bjorntorp, Metabolism of adipose tissue in intraabdominal depots of nonobese men and women. *Metabolism* 38, 453-458 (1989); published online EpubMay.

[63] B. B. Kahn, J. S. Flier, Obesity and insulin resistance. *J Clin Invest* 106, 473-481 (2000); published online EpubAug.

[64] J. Hellmer, C. Marcus, T. Sonnenfeld, P. Arner, Mechanisms for differences in lipolysis between human subcutaneous and omental fat cells. *J Clin Endocrinol Metab* 75, 15-20 (1992); published online EpubJul.

[65] P. Arner, L. Hellstrom, H. Wahrenberg, M. Bronnegard, Beta-adrenoceptor expression in human fat cells from different regions. *J Clin Invest* 86, 1595-1600 (1990); published online EpubNov.

[66] J. Bolinder, L. Kager, J. Ostman, P. Arner, Differences at the receptor and postreceptor levels between human omental and subcutaneous adipose tissue in the action of insulin on lipolysis. *Diabetes* 32, 117-123 (1983); published online EpubFeb.

[67] J. R. Zierath, J. N. Livingston, A. Thorne, J. Bolinder, S. Reynisdottir, F. Lonnqvist, P. Arner, Regional difference in insulin inhibition of non-esterified fatty acid release from human adipocytes: relation to insulin receptor phosphorylation and intracellular signalling through the insulin receptor substrate-1 pathway. *Diabetologia* 41, 1343-1354 (1998); published online EpubNov.

[68] J. B. Albu, M. Curi, M. Shur, L. Murphy, D. E. Matthews, F. X. Pi-Sunyer, Systemic resistance to the antilipolytic effect of insulin in black and white women with visceral obesity. *Am J Physiol* 277, E551-560 (1999); published online EpubSep.

[69] A. M. Lefebvre, M. Laville, N. Vega, J. P. Riou, L. van Gaal, J. Auwerx, H. Vidal, Depot-specific differences in adipose tissue gene expression in lean and obese subjects. *Diabetes* 47, 98-103 (1998); published online EpubJan.

[70] C. U. Niesler, K. Siddle, J. B. Prins, Human preadipocytes display a depot-specific susceptibility to apoptosis. *Diabetes* 47, 1365-1368 (1998); published online EpubAug.

[71] C. T. Montague, J. B. Prins, L. Sanders, J. Zhang, C. P. Sewter, J. Digby, C. D. Byrne, S. O'Rahilly, Depot-related gene expression in human subcutaneous and omental adipocytes. *Diabetes* 47, 1384-1391 (1998); published online EpubSep.

[72] H. Hauner, M. Wabitsch, E. F. Pfeiffer, Differentiation of adipocyte precursor cells from obese and nonobese adult women and from different adipose tissue sites. *Horm Metab Res Suppl* 19, 35-39 (1988).

[73] C. T. Montague, J. B. Prins, L. Sanders, J. E. Digby, S. O'Rahilly, Depot- and sex-specific differences in human leptin mRNA expression: implications for the control of regional fat distribution. *Diabetes* 46, 342-347 (1997); published online EpubMar.

[74] K. Samaras, N. K. Botelho, D. J. Chisholm, R. V. Lord, Subcutaneous and visceral adipose tissue gene expression of serum adipokines that predict type 2 diabetes. *Obesity (Silver Spring)* 18, 884-889 (2010); published online EpubMay (10.1038/oby.2009.443).

[75] J. N. Fain, A. K. Madan, M. L. Hiler, P. Cheema, S. W. Bahouth, Comparison of the release of adipokines by adipose tissue, adipose tissue matrix, and adipocytes from visceral and subcutaneous abdominal adipose tissues of obese humans. *Endocrinology* 145, 2273-2282 (2004); published online EpubMay (10.1210/en.2003-1336).

[76] V. Van Harmelen, S. Reynisdottir, P. Eriksson, A. Thorne, J. Hoffstedt, F. Lonnqvist, P. Arner, Leptin secretion from subcutaneous and visceral adipose tissue in women. *Diabetes* 47, 913-917 (1998); published online EpubJun.

[77] S. Baglioni, G. Cantini, G. Poli, M. Francalanci, R. Squecco, A. Di Franco, E. Borgogni, S. Frontera, G. Nesi, F. Liotta, M. Lucchese, G. Perigli, F. Francini, G. Forti, M. Serio, M. Luconi, Functional differences in visceral and subcutaneous fat pads originate from differences in the adipose stem cell. *PloS one* 7, e36569 (2012)10.1371/journal.pone.0036569).

[78] M. S. Mirza, Obesity, Visceral Fat, and NAFLD: Querying the Role of Adipokines in the Progression of Nonalcoholic Fatty Liver Disease. *ISRN gastroenterology* 2011, 592404 (2011)10.5402/2011/592404).

[79] C. Poussin, D. Hall, K. Minehira, A. M. Galzin, D. Tarussio, B. Thorens, Different transcriptional control of metabolism and extracellular matrix in visceral and subcutaneous fat of obese and rimonabant treated mice. *PloS one* 3, e3385 (2008)10.1371/journal.pone.0003385).

[80] J. Hoffstedt, E. Arner, H. Wahrenberg, D. P. Andersson, V. Qvisth, P. Lofgren, M. Ryden, A. Thorne, M. Wiren, M. Palmer, A. Thorell, E.

Toft, P. Arner, Regional impact of adipose tissue morphology on the metabolic profile in morbid obesity. *Diabetologia* 53, 2496-2503 (2010); published online EpubDec (10.1007/s00125-010-1889-3).

[81] O. Gealekman, N. Guseva, C. Hartigan, S. Apotheker, M. Gorgoglione, K. Gurav, K. V. Tran, J. Straubhaar, S. Nicoloro, M. P. Czech, M. Thompson, R. A. Perugini, S. Corvera, Depot-specific differences and insufficient subcutaneous adipose tissue angiogenesis in human obesity. *Circulation* 123, 186-194 (2011); published online EpubJan 18 (10.1161/CIRCULATIONAHA.110.970145).

[82] G. E. Alvarez, S. D. Beske, T. P. Ballard, K. P. Davy, Sympathetic neural activation in visceral obesity. *Circulation* 106, 2533-2536 (2002); published online EpubNov 12.

[83] A. Thorne, F. Lonnqvist, J. Apelman, G. Hellers, P. Arner, A pilot study of long-term effects of a novel obesity treatment: omentectomy in connection with adjustable gastric banding. *Int J Obes Relat Metab Disord* 26, 193-199 (2002); published online EpubFeb.

[84] F. Q. Milleo, A. C. Campos, S. Santoro, A. Lacombe, M. A. Santo, M. R. Vicari, V. Nogaroto, R. F. Artoni, Metabolic effects of an entero-omentectomy in mildly obese type 2 diabetes mellitus patients after three years. *Clinics* 66, 1227-1233 (2011).

[85] E. Fabbrini, R. A. Tamboli, F. Magkos, P. A. Marks-Shulman, A. W. Eckhauser, W. O. Richards, S. Klein, N. N. Abumrad, Surgical removal of omental fat does not improve insulin sensitivity and cardiovascular risk factors in obese adults. *Gastroenterology* 139, 448-455 (2010); published online EpubAug (10.1053/j.gastro.2010.04.056).

[86] M. F. Herrera, J. P. Pantoja, D. Velazquez-Fernandez, J. Cabiedes, C. Aguilar-Salinas, E. Garcia-Garcia, A. Rivas, C. Villeda, D. F. Hernandez-Ramirez, A. Davila, A. Zarain, Potential additional effect of omentectomy on metabolic syndrome, acute-phase reactants, and inflammatory mediators in grade III obese patients undergoing laparoscopic Roux-en-Y gastric bypass: a randomized trial. *Diabetes Care* 33, 1413-1418 (2010); published online EpubJul (10.2337/dc09-1833).

[87] N. Barzilai, L. She, B. Q. Liu, P. Vuguin, P. Cohen, J. Wang, L. Rossetti, Surgical removal of visceral fat reverses hepatic insulin resistance. *Diabetes* 48, 94-98 (1999); published online EpubJan.

[88] I. Gabriely, X. H. Ma, X. M. Yang, G. Atzmon, M. W. Rajala, A. H. Berg, P. Scherer, L. Rossetti, N. Barzilai, Removal of visceral fat prevents insulin resistance and glucose intolerance of aging: an

adipokine-mediated process? *Diabetes* 51, 2951-2958 (2002); published online EpubOct.

[89]   Y. W. Kim, J. Y. Kim, S. K. Lee, Surgical removal of visceral fat decreases plasma free fatty acid and increases insulin sensitivity on liver and peripheral tissue in monosodium glutamate (MSG)-obese rats. *J Korean Med Sci* 14, 539-545 (1999); published online EpubOct.

[90]   C. Pitombo, E. P. Araujo, C. T. De Souza, J. C. Pareja, B. Geloneze, L. A. Velloso, Amelioration of diet-induced diabetes mellitus by removal of visceral fat. *The Journal of endocrinology* 191, 699-706 (2006); published online EpubDec (10.1677/joe.1.07069).

[91]   M. T. Foster, H. Shi, R. J. Seeley, S. C. Woods, Transplantation or removal of intra-abdominal adipose tissue prevents age-induced glucose insensitivity. *Physiol Behav* 101, 282-288; published online EpubSep 1.

[92]   H. Shi, A. D. Strader, S. C. Woods, R. J. Seeley, The effect of fat removal on glucose tolerance is depot specific in male and female mice. *American journal of physiology. Endocrinology and metabolism* 293, E1012-1020 (2007); published online EpubOct (10.1152/ajpendo. 00649.2006).

[93]   R. B. Harris, R. L. Leibel, Location, location, location. *Cell Metab* 7, 359-361 (2008); published online EpubMay.

[94]   M. T. Foster, H. Shi, R. J. Seeley, S. C. Woods, Removal of intra-abdominal visceral adipose tissue improves glucose tolerance in rats: role of hepatic triglyceride storage. *Physiol Behav* 104, 845-854 (2011); published online EpubOct 24 (S0031-9384(11)00298-8 [pii] 10.1016/j.physbeh.2011.04.064).

[95]   A. B. Arie, L. McNally, D. S. Kapp, N. N. H. Teng, The omentum and omentectomy in epithelial ovarian cancer: A reappraisal: Part II — The role of omentectomy in the staging and treatment of apparent early stage epithelial ovarian cancer. *Gynecologic Oncology* 131, 784-790 (2013); published online Epub12// (http://dx.doi.org/10.1016 /j.ygyno.2013.09.013).

[96]   R. K. Jan Hauspy, and Allan L. Covens, in *Laparoscopic Surgery for Gynecologic Oncology*. (McGraw Hill, 2008), chap. Miscellaneous, including Omentectomy, Appendectomy, Lysis, Adhesions, and Splenectomy, pp. 143-155.

[97]   M.-C. Kim, K.-H. Kim, G. J. Jung, D. W. Rattner, Comparative Study of Complete and Partial Omentectomy in Radical Subtotal Gastrectomy for Early Gastric Cancer. *Yonsei Med J* 52, 961-966 (2011); published online Epub11.

[98] M. Alagumuthu, B. B. Das, S. P. Pattanayak, M. Rasananda, The omentum: A unique organ of exceptional versatility. *Indian Journal of Surgery* 68, 136-141 (2006).

[99] R. E. Mebius, Lymphoid Organs for Peritoneal Cavity Immune Response: Milky Spots. *Immunity* 30, 670-672 (2009); published online Epub5/22/ (http://dx.doi.org/10.1016/j.immuni.2009.04.005).

[100] C. L. Willard-Mack, Normal Structure, Function, and Histology of Lymph Nodes. *Toxicologic Pathology* 34, 409-424 (2006); published online EpubAugust 1, 2006 (10.1080/01926230600867727).

[101] A. Yildirim, A. Aktas, Y. Nergiz, M. Akkus, Analysis of human omentum-associated lymphoid tissue components with S-100: an immunohistochemical study. *Romanian journal of morphology and embryology = Revue roumaine de morphologie et embryologie* 51, 759-764 (2010).

[102] D. C. Cameron Platell, John M. Papadimitriou, and John C. hall, The Omentum. *World Journal of Gastroenterology* 6, 169-176 (2000); published online EpubApril, 2000.

[103] L. F. G. Krist, I. L. Eestermans, J. J. E. Steenbergen, E. C. M. Hoefsmit, M. A. Cuesta, S. Meyer, R. H. J. Beelen, Cellular composition of milky spots in the human greater omentum: An immunochemical and ultrastructural study. *The Anatomical Record* 241, 163-174 (1995)10.1002/ar.1092410204).

[104] J. F. Wijffels, R. J. Hendrickx, J. J. Steenbergen, I. L. Eestermans, R. H. Beelen, Milky spots in the mouse omentum may play an important role in the origin of peritoneal macrophages. *Research in immunology* 143, 401-409 (1992); published online EpubMay.

[105] C. Hodel, Ultrastructural studies on the absorption of protein markers by the greater omentum. *European surgical research. Europaische chirurgische Forschung. Recherches chirurgicales europeennes* 2, 435-449 (1970).

[106] E. Mandache, E. Moldoveanu, G. Savi, The involvement of omentum and its milky spots in the dynamics of peritoneal macrophages. *Morphologie et embryologie* 31, 137-142 (1985); published online EpubApr-Jun.

[107] H. F. Dullens, L. H. Rademakers, S. Cluistra, R. Van Os, K. Dux, P. J. Den Besten, W. Den Otter, Parathymic lymph nodes during growth and rejection of intraperitoneally inoculated tumor cells. *Invasion & metastasis* 11, 216-226 (1991).

[108] J. Rangel-Moreno, J. E. Moyron-Quiroz, D. M. Carragher, K. Kusser, L. Hartson, A. Moquin, T. D. Randall, Omental milky spots develop in the absence of lymphoid tissue-inducer cells and support B and T cell responses to peritoneal antigens. *Immunity* 30, 731-743 (2009); published online EpubMay (10.1016/j.immuni.2009.03.014).

[109] C. M. Pond, C. A. Mattacks, In vivo evidence for the involvement of the adipose tissue surrounding lymph nodes in immune responses. *Immunology Letters* 63, 159-167 (1998); published online Epub10// (http://dx.doi.org/10.1016/S0165-2478(98)00074-1).

[110] C. M. Pond, Adipose tissue and the immune system. *Prostaglandins, Leukotrienes and Essential Fatty Acids* 73, 17-30 (2005); published online Epub7// (http://dx.doi.org/10.1016/j.plefa.2005.04.005).

[111] N. L. Harvey, The Link between Lymphatic Function and Adipose Biology. *Annals of the New York Academy of Sciences* 1131, 82-88 (2008)10.1196/annals.1413.007).

[112] D. Sadler, C. A. Mattacks, C. M. Pond, Changes in adipocytes and dendritic cells in lymph node containing adipose depots during and after many weeks of mild inflammation. *Journal of Anatomy* 207, 769-781 (2005)10.1111/j.1469-7580.2005.00506.x).

[113] R. M. Steinman, The Dendritic Cell System and its Role in Immunogenicity. *Annual Review of Immunology* 9, 271-296 (1991); published online Epub1991/04/01 (10.1146/annurev.iy.09.040191.001415).

[114] C. A. Mattacks, D. Sadler, C. M. Pond, The cellular structure and lipid/protein composition of adipose tissue surrounding chronically stimulated lymph nodes in rats. *J Anat* 202, 551-561 (2003); published online EpubJun.

[115] J. Nougues, Y. Reyne, J. P. Dulor, Differentiation of rabbit adipocyte precursors in primary culture. *Int J Obes* 12, 321-333 (1988).

[116] N. L. Harvey, R. S. Srinivasan, M. E. Dillard, N. C. Johnson, M. H. Witte, K. Boyd, M. W. Sleeman, G. Oliver, Lymphatic vascular defects promoted by Prox1 haploinsufficiency cause adult-onset obesity. *Nature genetics* 37, 1072-1081 (2005); published online EpubOct (10.1038/ng1642).

[117] H. Brorson, Liposuction in arm lymphedema treatment. *Scandinavian journal of surgery : SJS : official organ for the Finnish Surgical Society and the Scandinavian Surgical Society* 92, 287-295 (2003).

[118] S. Shah, E. Lowery, R. K. Braun, A. Martin, N. Huang, M. Medina, P. Sethupathi, Y. Seki, M. Takami, K. Byrne, C. Wigfield, R. B. Love, M.

Iwashima, Cellular Basis of Tissue Regeneration by Omentum. *PloS one* 7, e38368 (2012)10.1371/journal.pone.0038368).

[119] B. Thakur, C. S. Zhang, Z. B. Tan, Omentoplasty versus no omentoplasty for esophagogastrostomy after surgery for cancer of cardia and esophagus. *Indian journal of cancer* 41, 167-169 (2004); published online EpubOct-Dec.

[120] H. Rafael, R. Mego, P. Moromizato, W. Garcia, Omental transplantation for temporal lobe epilepsy: report of two cases. *Neurology India* 50, 71-74 (2002); published online EpubMar.

[121] T. Krabatsch, D. V. Schmitt, F. W. Mohr, R. Hetzer, Thoracic transposition of the greater omentum as an adjunct in the treatment of mediastinitis--pros and cons within the context of a randomised study. *The European journal of surgery. Supplement. : = Acta chirurgica. Supplement*, 45-48 (1999).

[122] J. F. Kusiak, N. G. Rosenblum, Neovaginal reconstruction after exenteration using an omental flap and split-thickness skin graft. *Plastic and reconstructive surgery* 97, 775-781; discussion 783-773 (1996); published online EpubApr.

[123] G. Ogunc, Minilaparoscopic extraperitoneal tunneling with omentopexy: a new technique for CAPD catheter placement. *Peritoneal dialysis international : journal of the International Society for Peritoneal Dialysis* 25, 551-555 (2005); published online EpubNov-Dec.

[124] N. J. de Wit, H. Bosch-Vermeulen, P. J. de Groot, G. J. Hooiveld, M. M. Bromhaar, J. Jansen, M. Muller, R. van der Meer, The role of the small intestine in the development of dietary fat-induced obesity and insulin resistance in C57BL/6J mice. *BMC medical genomics* 1, 14 (2008)10.1186/1755-8794-1-14).

[125] T. F. Teixeira, M. C. Collado, C. L. Ferreira, J. Bressan, C. Peluzio Mdo, Potential mechanisms for the emerging link between obesity and increased intestinal permeability. *Nutrition research* 32, 637-647 (2012); published online EpubSep (10.1016/j.nutres.2012.07.003).

[126] H. Wu, S. Ghosh, X. D. Perrard, L. Feng, G. E. Garcia, J. L. Perrard, J. F. Sweeney, L. E. Peterson, L. Chan, C. W. Smith, C. M. Ballantyne, T-cell accumulation and regulated on activation, normal T cell expressed and secreted upregulation in adipose tissue in obesity. *Circulation* 115, 1029-1038 (2007); published online EpubFeb 27 (10.1161/CIRCULATIONAHA.106.638379).

[127] U. Kintscher, M. Hartge, K. Hess, A. Foryst-Ludwig, M. Clemenz, M. Wabitsch, P. Fischer-Posovszky, T. F. Barth, D. Dragun, T. Skurk, H.

Hauner, M. Bluher, T. Unger, A. M. Wolf, U. Knippschild, V. Hombach, N. Marx, T-lymphocyte infiltration in visceral adipose tissue: a primary event in adipose tissue inflammation and the development of obesity-mediated insulin resistance. *Arteriosclerosis, thrombosis, and vascular biology* 28, 1304-1310 (2008); published online EpubJul (10.1161/ATVBAHA.108.165100).

[128] M. M. Altintas, A. Azad, B. Nayer, G. Contreras, J. Zaias, C. Faul, J. Reiser, A. Nayer, Mast cells, macrophages, and crown-like structures distinguish subcutaneous from visceral fat in mice. *Journal of lipid research* 52, 480-488 (2011); published online EpubMar (10.1194/jlr.M011338).

[129] J. Deiuliis, Z. Shah, N. Shah, B. Needleman, D. Mikami, V. Narula, K. Perry, J. Hazey, T. Kampfrath, M. Kollengode, Q. Sun, A. R. Satoskar, C. Lumeng, S. Moffatt-Bruce, S. Rajagopalan, Visceral adipose inflammation in obesity is associated with critical alterations in tregulatory cell numbers. *PloS one* 6, e16376 (2011)10.1371 /journal.pone.0016376).

[130] J. B. McLachlan, J. P. Hart, S. V. Pizzo, C. P. Shelburne, H. F. Staats, M. D. Gunn, S. N. Abraham, Mast cell-derived tumor necrosis factor induces hypertrophy of draining lymph nodes during infection. *Nature immunology* 4, 1199-1205 (2003); published online EpubDec (10.1038/ni1005).

[131] H. W. Wang, N. Tedla, A. R. Lloyd, D. Wakefield, P. H. McNeil, Mast cell activation and migration to lymph nodes during induction of an immune response in mice. *J Clin Invest* 102, 1617-1626 (1998); published online EpubOct 15 (10.1172/JCI3704).

[132] C. S. Kim, S. C. Lee, Y. M. Kim, B. S. Kim, H. S. Choi, T. Kawada, B. S. Kwon, R. Yu, Visceral fat accumulation induced by a high-fat diet causes the atrophy of mesenteric lymph nodes in obese mice. *Obesity (Silver Spring)* 16, 1261-1269 (2008); published online EpubJun (10.1038/oby.2008.55).

[133] M. R. Gibbs, L. B. Pemberton, N. J. Litton, W. R. Snider, Lipolymph nodes of the mesentery. *The American surgeon* 51, 596-598 (1985); published online EpubOct.

In: General and Abdominal Surgery
Editor: Kassandra Sarah Slavomir

ISBN: 978-1-63117-440-7
© 2014 Nova Science Publishers, Inc.

Chapter 2

Bariatric Surgery:
Indications and Complications

***Dina M. Filiberto and Aziz M. Merchant**[*]*
Rutgers–New Jersey Medical School, Department of Surgery

Abstract

Bariatric surgery has become a mainstay in the treatment armamentarium of morbid obesity. Randomized trials have established the efficacy of bariatric surgery towards sustained weight loss, along with significant improvements in related comorbidities, quality of life measures, and all-cause mortality. The most commonly performed and effective procedures include the Laparoscopic Roux-en-Y gastric bypass (LRYGBP), Laparoscopic adjustable gastric banding (LAGB), and Laparoscopic sleeve gastrectomy (LSG). Minimally invasive approaches have become the standard of care as they are associated with smaller incisions, less post-operative pain, fewer respiratory complications, and fewer wound complications.

As with any complex surgical procedure, there are significant complications associated with these operations, including incisional hernias, deep vein thromboses, pulmonary emboli, wound infections, anastomotic leaks, bleeding, and intestinal obstruction. Procedure-

[*] Corresponding author: Aziz M. Merchant, MD FACS, Rutgers–New Jersey Medical School, Department of Surgery, 185 South Orange Street Suite MSB G514, Newark, NJ 07103, Tel No.: (973) 972-2205 (Office), (973) 972-6803 (Fax), Email: Aziz.Merchant@Rutgers.edu.

specific complications include band slippage, band erosion, internal hernias, dumping syndrome, vitamin deficiencies, marginal ulcers, strictures, and esophageal reflux. Post-operative care in patients with failure of the initial procedure or with complications is challenging and may necessitate revision and reoperation. We present a brief review of bariatric surgical procedures, discussion of potential complications, and accepted management of these complications.

Introduction

Obesity is a continued problem in the United States, with a prevalence of 35% in the adult population [1]. It is associated with multiple comorbidities such as diabetes, obstructive sleep apnea, and cardiovascular disease. According to the NIH, patients with a BMI > 40, or those with a BMI >35 and < 40 with high-risk comorbid conditions, are considered candidates for surgery [2]. Bariatric surgery has been shown to produce sustained weight loss and improvement in these comorbidities. The procedures themselves have undergone repetitive refinement over the years, and with the introduction of laparoscopy, patients have had improved outcomes and fewer complications. Laparoscopic Roux-en-Y gastric bypass (LRYGB), Laparoscopic adjustable gastric banding (LAGB), and Laparoscopic sleeve gastrectomy (LSG) are the most commonly performed bariatric procedures today [3]. Morbidity in bariatric surgery, although quite low in overall rates, can be devastating due to the high-risk profile of these patients and the nature and complexity of the operations. A high index of suspicion, along with timely identification and management of complications is paramount for success.

Review of Bariatric Procedures

Laparoscopic ROUX-EN-Y Gastric Bypass

The RYGB is the most common bariatric procedure performed in the world, and is considered the gold standard for bariatric surgery [3]. The operation results in weight loss by gastric restriction and intestinal malabsorption. There is increasing evidence that a metabolic component plays a role in appetite and eating behavior postoperatively, secondary to the changes in circulating levels of gastrointestinal hormones, such as ghrelin and

PYY [4]. In most bariatric procedures, typically five to six laparoscopic ports are used in the upper abdomen, with standard carbon dioxide insufflation. A number of modifications of standard technique exist, however the basics are presented here. The liver is retracted upward to reveal the gastroesophageal junction anatomy. A gastric pouch is created by transection with a linear stapler across the lesser curvature of the stomach 3 to 5 cm distal to the gastroesophageal junction to create the 15 to 30 mL volume pouch. The biliopancreatic limb is measured to approximately 50-80cm, and a Roux-limb of about 75-150 cm is established with a stapled side-to-side, functional end-to-end jejunojejunostomy. A gastrojejunostomy is then created using a 21 or 25-mm end-to-end anastomosis (EEA) circular stapler, linear stapler, or hand sewn technique [5]. The roux limb may be brought up to the gastric pouch in a retrocolic and retrogastric, or antecolic and antegastric, fashion. The mesenteric defect of the jejunojejunostomy may be closed based on operating surgeon preference. Another optional aspect of the operation is a leak test for the gastrojejunostomy, which may be performed via instillation of methylene blue or air through an orogastric tube or by upper endoscopy [6].

Laparoscopic Adjustable Gastric Band

The LAGB involves placement of a silicone band with an adjustable balloon around the proximal stomach. Weight loss is the result of gastric restriction by the band. The band is attached by inert tubing to an injectable single-access port which is placed in the subcutaneous tissue and anchored to the fascia of the abdominal wall. The port site is accessible by needle access through skin and subcutaneous tissue. There are two techniques of dissection to access the retrogastric space to deliver the band. The perigastric technique involves dissection between the wall of the stomach and blood supply high on the lesser curvature. The lesser sac is entered, and dissection continues to the omental bursalis, and the gastric band is placed encircling the stomach at this area. The pars flaccida technique minimizes perigastric dissection. The phrenoesophageal ligament at the angle of His is entered and the gastrohepatic ligament is taken down. The retroperitoneum at the posterior extension of the right crus is incised and dissected retrogastric to the angle of His. The band is placed at this location. Gastric plication with interrupted sutures may be performed to secure the position of the band. One may place a stitch in the anterior gastric wall inferior to the band to prevent slippage [6]. The tubing is tunneled through the subcutaneous tissue to the desired port site and attached to the access port. The access port is then placed on the abdominal wall fascia. Postoperatively, the band is filled with fluid in the office or in a radiologic suite under fluoroscopy. Intermittent adjustments are made to the band volume so the patient loses 1 to 2 pounds per week.

Laparoscopic Sleeve Gastrectomy

The LSG is a newer procedure, being performed with increasing frequency. It was originally performed as the first part of a staged approach to super-morbidly obese patients, followed by a biliopancreatic diversion with duodenal switch or a Roux-en-y gastric bypass. As results looked promising for long-term effective weight loss and comorbidity resolution, it eventually became a stand-alone procedure [7]. Proponents of the LSG tout its advantages compared to the LRYGB, as it is simpler in technique and purely restrictive, resulting in fewer of the vitamin and protein deficiencies seen in malabsorptive procedures. The short gastric and epicardial vessels are ligated from the angle of His to several centimeters shy of the pylorus, mobilizing the greater curvature of the stomach. The sleeve remnant is sized with a bougie or an endoscope, and approximately 85% of the stomach is then excluded using a linear stapler, beginning 5 to 7cm proximal to the pylorus. The gastric remnant is removed and the staple line may be oversewn [5]. A staple-line leak test may be performed using air or methylene blue in the orogastric tube or endoscope [6].

Complications

Mortality

Decades of experience with bariatric surgery have produced perioperative and intraoperative refinements to patient care resulting in an impressive track record of patient safety. Morino published an analysis, from a 10-year prospectively collected database, of over 13,000 bariatric procedures where the 60-day mortality was 0.25%. Subcategory analysis showed that the mortality for LAGB and LRYGB was 0.08% and 0.58%, respectively. This rate is comparable to that of elective incisional hernia repairs (0.5%), and better than that of elective colon resections (1.5%) [8, 9]. The most common causes of death were pulmonary embolus, cardiac failure, anastomotic leak, and other causes of respiratory failure. Risk factors for mortality included open surgery, increased operative time, pre-operative hypertension and diabetes, and low hospital bariatric case volume [10].

Similarly, Flum reviewed prospectively collected data in 4,776 patients undergoing bariatric procedures from 2005 to 2007 and found the 30-day mortality to be 0.3%. LRYGB comprised 62% these procedures, followed by LAGB with 25.1%, and open RYGB making up 9%. The mortality ranged from zero in those who underwent LAGB, to 0.2% in LRYGB, to 2.1% in open RYGB. Patients with a higher BMI, poor functional status, history of venous thromboembolism (VTE), or history of obstructive sleep apnea had worse outcomes [11]. A more recent prospective, observational analysis by Hutter, using data from over 100 programs and 28,000 patients who had LAGB, LSG, LRYGB, and open RYGB, showed an overall mortality of 0.12%. Open RYGB was the only procedure with a significantly higher mortality of 0.71% [12]. This evidence clearly demonstrates a consistent low mortality rate of laparoscopic bariatric procedures.

Common Post-Operative Complications

Wound Infections and Incisional Hernias

Obesity has been found to be an independent risk factor for surgical site infection in general surgery literature. Clearly relevant to the bariatric surgical population, a recent meta-analysis reviewed laparoscopic versus open surgical procedures in obese patients and their impact on wound infections. There was a 70-80% lower risk of surgical site infection after laparoscopic surgery than after open surgery [13]. Nguyen published a randomized trial between open and laparoscopic RYGB, and found wound-related complications were higher in the open group as compared to the laparoscopic group (10.5% vs 1.3%), as was the incidence of incisional hernias (7.9% vs 0%) after 1 year follow up. In the one patient who developed a wound infection at the port site in the laparoscopic group, local wound care and oral antibiotics were sufficient treatment, however all of the patients in the open group with wound infection required open drainage and a prolonged course of wound care [14].

Venous Thromboembolism

VTE is an uncommon, but potentially fatal complication following bariatric surgery. Using data from a large longitudinal database, Winegar reported the risk of VTE within 90 days of surgery was 0.42%. Risk of VTE was greater in those undergoing RYGB versus LAGB, and was also associated with open surgery, age, higher BMI, and history of VTE [15]. Stein found that following bariatric surgery, the prevalence of pulmonary embolus or DVT was 2.2%. In hospital death was 0.03% among those with VTE [16]. There are no specific recommendations for VTE prophylaxis in bariatric surgery. For those undergoing abdominal surgery the American College of Chest physicians recommends pharmacologic prophylaxis or mechanical prophylaxis, and sometimes both [17].

Bleeding

The cause for gastrointestinal bleeding (GIB) after LRGYB and LSG is usually related to the staple lines. The long staple line of the LSG poses a significant risk. Silecchia reported staple-line bleeding in 7.3% of patients who underwent LSG in a prospective study [18]. Mittermair found a postoperative bleeding rate of 3.3% all of which required re-laparoscopy. Patients presented with typical signs and symptoms of GIB; tachycardia, decrease in hemoglobin, melena, hypotension [19].

Incidence of GIB after LRYGB is reported between 1.1% and 4% [20]. Early presentation of postoperative bleeding (<48 hours) consists of hematemesis, bright red blood per rectum, hypotension, tachycardia and decreasing hemoglobin, and usually necessitates intervention. Late presentation (>48 hours) consists of melena, and may or may not be accompanied by change in vital signs and decreased hemoglobin. This subgroup of patients may often be managed conservatively [20]. Upper endoscopy is most successful in patients with hemorrhage from the gastric pouch or gastrojejunostomy. Those with hematemesis and bright blood per rectum in the setting of clinical signs of bleeding require operative intervention by laparoscopic or open approach. If the bypassed stomach is distended, a gastrotomy can be performed for decompression, and all staple-lines must be oversewn [21].

Procedure Specific Complications

Roux-en-Y Gastric Bypass

Anastomotic Leak

The Achilles heel of the gold standard bariatric operation, the RYGB, is the anastomotic leak, a potentially life-threatening complication with high morbidity and mortality. The rate of anastomotic leak is reported to be 1-5%, with similar rates among open and laparoscopic procedures. Fernandez performed a prospective study of more than 3,000 patients who underwent LRYGB and open RYGB, the overall incidence of leak was 3.2%. Significant risk factors were diabetes and obstructive sleep apnea. The overall mortality in this series was 1.5%, and leak was associated with 16.7% of these patients [22]. Anastomotic leak is the second leading cause of death in patients who undergo RYGB. The site of anastomotic leak is most commonly the gastrojejunostomy (69% in one study by Ballesta) however, it can also occur at the gastric pouch or remnant staple lines, and the jejunojejunostomy. Technical or operative risk factors for anastomotic leaks include tension on the anastomosis, staple or stapler malfunction, surgical technique, obstruction and ischemia [23]. Patient factors for leak include the presence of multiple co-morbidities such as hypertension, diabetes, obstructive sleep apnea, BMI, age, venous insufficiency, and reoperative surgery [24].

Diagnosis requires experience and a high index of suspicion, especially in those who do not progress as expected during the first postoperative day. Signs and symptoms include worsening abdominal pain, nausea, tachypnea, fever, tachycardia, hypotension and oliguria [23,24]. Yet up to 50% of patients with anastomotic leak may be asymptomatic, with the only indication of leak being abnormal output in the patients drain, and leak confirmed with oral methylene blue test[24]. Other diagnostic studies used to confirm anastomotic leak include an upper gastrointestinal (UGI) series and an oral contrast-enhanced computer tomographic (CT) scan, in patients who are stable. However, in the unstable patient with signs and symptoms of worsening sepsis, the next most important step may be to forego the study in favor of immediate operative intervention.

Treatment is comprised of appropriate resuscitation, adequate drainage, complete control of sepsis, antibiotics, and nutritional support either enterally or parenterally. If the patient is clinically stable, a cautious, vigilant trial of conservative management may be warranted with IV antibiotics, drain monitoring, and parenteral nutrition. This was shown to be successful in 35 out of 36 patients in a retrospective analysis of patients with anastomotic leak [24]. Patients that are hemodynamically unstable with complicated leaks and signs of sepsis, should undergo immediate operative treatment, with wide drainage, repair or patching of the defect indicated, and possible placement of feeding gastrostomy. Ballesta performed a retrospective review of 1,200 patients who underwent LRYGB, and of 59 patients with anastomotic leak, 38% underwent operative treatment. Late sequelae occurred in 35% including gastrojejunal strictures, gastrogastric fistulas, anastomotic ulcers, and obstruction [24].

Stricture

The incidence of gastrojejunostomy stricture after LRYGB ranges from 3-27%[25,26]. Common presentation is intolerance to solid food with progression to intolerance to liquids, nausea, and emesis. Strictures may present weeks to months after surgery, sometimes even years out. The etiology of stricture is thought to be due ischemia, marginal ulceration, anastomotic leak with scar formation, or technical error. The route of the roux limb (antecolic versus retrocolic) and surgical approach (laparoscopic versus open) has produced comparable stricture rates [25,26,27]. However, there is evidence that the method of construction of the gastrojejunostomy may have a role in the occurrence of a stricture. Use of a linear stapler results in stricture rate of 3.1% to 6.8% [26,27,28] versus the use of a 21-mm circular stapler, which results in stricture rates of 15.5% to 17% [29,30]. This rate was reduced to 8.8% and 6.2% with use of the 25-mm circular stapler [29,31]. There may be discrepancy in the reporting of stricture rates due to the way surgeons define a stricture and how often symptomatic patients undergo diagnostic procedures.

Diagnosis can be made with barium swallow, which may show a distal narrowing, or upper endoscopy, which will give visual, intraluminal confirmation. Moreover, flexible upper endoscopy can help determine the severity of the stricture, delineate anatomy, identify potential causes, allow a tissue diagnosis, and allow symptomatic relief through dilatation. According to Go, endoscopic dilation is a successful treatment strategy, with an average amount of dilations ranging from 1.6 to 2.1 and a rare need for operative intervention [25,27]. The main complication associated with endoscopic dilation of an anastomotic stricture is perforation, with an incidence in the literature of 1.6% to 2.2% [25,26,28].

Marginal Ulcers

A marginal ulcer is a peptic ulcer near the site of the gastrojejunal anastomosis. The incidence varies in the literature from 3.5% to 7% [32,33,34]. Rasmussen found that *helicobacter pylori* infection was twice as common in those with marginal ulcers compared with those who were not affected [32]. Dallal prospectively studied 201 consecutive LRYGB procedures and found those with marginal ulceration presented with perforation, bleeding requiring transfusion or severe pain on average of 7.4

months postoperatively. Patients were successfully treated with proton pump inhibitors (PPIs) and sucralfate. There were no preoperative predictors of ulcer disease [33]. Gumbs prospectively studied 347 patients who underwent LRGYB, and found that those with marginal ulceration presented with abdominal pain and upper gastrointestinal bleeding 6.3 months postoperatively. Again resolution was seen in all patients after treatment with PPIs. Additionally, prophylactic PPIs were given postoperatively towards the end of the study period, and no patients subsequently developed marginal ulceration [34]. Azagury performed a retrospective study of patients with marginal ulcer at endoscopy and found 63% presented with pain and/or 24% presented with bleeding. Sutures were visible in 35% and gastrogastric fistulae were identified in 8%. Significant risk factors were diabetes, smoking and long gastric pouches, suggesting increased acid exposure and mucosal ischemia are involved in ulcer pathogenesis. In this series, 9% of patients required surgical revision. [35]

Dumping Syndrome

Dumping syndrome is a common complication of gastroesophageal surgery, which is also encountered after RYGB. The clinical presentation is variable and is usually divided into early and late dumping phases. Early dumping symptoms are attributed to the rapid transit of hyperosmotic chime into the jejunum resulting in fluid shifts and release of vasoactive substances [36]. Symptoms include flushing, dizziness, palpitations, abdominal pain, diarrhea, nausea, and bloating [36,37]. Late dumping symptoms usually occur 1-3 hours post-prandially, secondary to reactive hypoglycemia [37]. Symptoms include palpitations, sweating, tremor, irritability, and drowsiness [36]. Several scoring systems and questionnaires have been used to characterize dumping syndrome, and the incidence after RYGB varies in the literature from 15.7% to 76% [37,38]. Banerjee found that 57% of patients who complained of dumping syndrome, did so early, while the rest complained of both early and late dumping, and all the patients' symptoms resolved within two years post RYGB [39]. Managing dumping syndrome centers largely on dietary measures. Patients are advised to consume small, frequent, low glycemic meals throughout the day. In patients with refractory dumping syndrome, use of somatostatin anaologs has been shown to improve symptoms and quality of life. Arts demonstrated that short and long-acting octreotide significantly reduced dumping syndrome symptoms in all patients, and patient's evaluations of their overall treatment efficacy was higher in the long-acting octreotide group as compared with the short-acting octreotride group (83% vs 52%) [36].

Obstruction and Internal Hernia

LRYGB has many advantages over the open approach, however there is a higher incidence of small bowel obstruction in the literature (4-5% vs 1-3%)[40,41,42,43]. The most common causes of obstruction after LRYGB are internal hernia (42-61% of cases), adhesions, and jejunojejunostomy stenosis[41,42,43]. Technical aspects of the operation affect the incidence of internal hernia, including closure or non-closure of mesenteric defects and antecolic versus retrocolic roux limb position[44]. There are three sites where internal hernias occur. The retrocolic retrogastric approach creates the transverse mesocolon defect, the jejunojejunostomy defect, and the space between the mesentery of the roux limb and transverse mesocolon (Petersen's defect). The antecolic antegastric approach creates a jejunojejunosotmy defect and Petersen's defect [45]. Steele compared the antecolic versus retrocolic approach, with all mesenteric defects closed, and found an incidence of 2.6% versus 0% of internal hernias in the retrocolic and antecolic groups, respectively [46]. Obeid found that of 914 patients who underwent LRYGB, 5% developed a symptomatic internal hernia that required surgical intervention. The incidence was lower in the mesenteric closure group as compared to the non-closure group (3.8% vs 8.4%). The incidence was also lower in the antecolic versus retrocolic roux limb group (3.8% vs 8.5%). This evidence suggests an antecolic approach with closure of all mesenteric defects. In all series, the most common symptoms were postprandial abdominal pain, nausea and emesis [44,45]. CT scan was consistent with presence of an internal hernia in 57.5% of patients, however 17.8% of patients had negative CT scan finding s[44]. In patients without definitive findings on imaging, a diagnostic laparoscopy may be indicated [46].

Vitamin Deficiencies

Vitamin B12 and Folate

LRYGB induces weight loss by a combination of restriction and malabsorption. Due to the malabsorptive mechanism of weight loss, patients are at risk for developing nutritional deficiencies because of the reduction in absorptive capacity of the small bowel [47]. Ingested food and enzymes are only mixed in the common limb located in the distal ileum [48]. Deficiencies of vitamin B12 and folate can result in the development of anemia. Vitamin B12 is bound to protein and cleaved by gastric acid and pepsin in the stomach, it then binds to intrinsic factor and is absorbed in the terminal ileum [47]. In patients with RYGB, the stomach and duodenum are excluded and vitamin B12 deficiency occurs due to decreased gastric secretions and inadequate function of intrinsic factor[49]. Folic acid is absorbed primarily in the proximal third of the small bowel, and deficiency results from decreased dietary intake and reduction in absorption in the small intestine [48]. Consequences of vitamin B12 and folate deficiencies include macrocytic anemia, leukopenia, glossitis, thrombocytopenia, paresthesia, and neuropathies [49]. The prevalence of vitamin B12 deficiency is estimated at 12-37%, with clinical symptoms occurring less frequently [50,51,52]. Vitamin B12 and folate deficiencies are usually correctable with oral supplementation, and rarely require parenteral administration [47].

Thiamine

Thiamine is absorbed in the duodenum, and deficiency occurs through reduction of acid production, reduced dietary intake, and hyperemesis. Lakhani reported an incidence of thiamine deficiency up to 49%, and suggested small intestinal bacterial overgrowth may play increase the risk of thiamine deficiency [53]. A consequence of thiamine deficiency is Wernicke encephalopathy, characterized by ataxia, confusion, ophthalmoplegia, and has been seen in RYGB patients, albeit rarely [54]. Oral supplementation is recommended prophylactically, and parenteral administration may be given in malnourished patients [49].

Calcium and Vitamin D

Calcium and vitamin D are maximally absorbed in the duodenum and proximal jejunum, and because of their exclusion in RYGB patients, deficiencies are common and result in bone mass abnormalities. Calcium and vitamin D deficiencies stimulate hyperparathyroidism and long-term risk of osteoporosis [47]. Clements found vitamin D deficiency and hyperparathyroidism in 23% and 25.7% of LRYGB patients after one year, respectively [55]. Coates found elevation of bone-turnover markers in patients after LRYGB despite calcium and vitamin D supplementation and unchanged serum levels of vitamin D and parathyroid hormone. Nine months after surgery, bone mineral density was reduced in the hip, trochanter, and total body[56]. Again, oral supplementation is recommended.

Vitamins A, E, K

Lipid soluble vitamins A, E, and K, are all at risk for malabsorption due to small intestine anatomy after gastric bypass and decreased intake of dietary lipids. Vitamin A deficiency was found in 11% of patients despite oral supplementation [57]. Only case reports describe xeropthalmia and blindness from vitamin A deficiency in RYGB patients [58]. Research on vitamin K and vitamin E deficiencies in the bariatric literature is limited. Diniz found that 50% of RYGB patients had low vitamin K levels; however they did not exhibit any clotting abnormalities [59]. Most of the studies on vitamin E deficiency are secondary to biliopancreatic diversion, and none of the patients exhibited clinical manifestions [49].

Sleeve Gastrectomy

Staple Line Leak

The most feared and dangerous complication of the LSG is a staple line leak. The incidence ranges from 0.7% to 7% [60,61,62]. Parikh performed a systematic review and found the overall incidence of staple line leak was 2.2%. He determined there is an increased risk of staple line leak with bougie size less than 40 French, and found that buttressing the staple line had no effect on leak, nor did staple line distance from the pylorus [63]. In a comparison of LSG with and without staple line reinforcement, there was no difference found in leak rate, as well as other parameters including bleeding and return to operation, by Merchant, et al. [64]. Aurora found that in 29 publications analyzed, there was a significantly higher leak rate of 3% in the super-obese population. He also found that a bougie less than 40 French was associated with increased leak rate. Location of the leak occurs primarily at the proximal portion of the staple-line, with 89% of documented leaks at the esophagogastric junction. Additionally, of the leaks with documented time of diagnosis, 79% occurred more than 10 days postoperatively [62].

In most patients, diagnosis was made after UGI series. Treatment options include conservative management (NPO/intravenous antibiotics/total parenteral nutrition), stent placement, percutaneous drainage and surgical revision or debridement [62,65].

Reflux

There is inconsistent data on the effect of LSG on gastroesophageal reflux (GER) symptoms. Symptomatic GER has been reported in 7.8-20% of patients after LSG [66,67,68,69]. Himpens retrospectively analyzed long-term effects and side effects of LSG, and found that 21% of patients developed GER symptoms after the third postoperative year [69]. Daes evaluated technical aspects of the LSG, and concluded that despite high preoperative incidence of GER (49%) and hiatal hernia (25.3%), careful surgical technique including repair of the hiatal hernia, and avoiding dilation of the fundus and narrowing of the junction of the sleeve, can result in a low incidence of GER postoperatively (1.5%) [70]. Further studies are necessary to sufficiently draw conclusions regarding GER after LSG.

Stricture

Incidence of stricture of the gastric sleeve after LSG ranges from 0.5% to 4% [60,62]. Typical symptoms include dysphagia, vomiting, and rapid weight loss [71]. A retrospective study by Parikh found that 3.5% of patients had a symptomatic stricture, with diagnosis confirmed by either contrast study (71%) or endoscopy (100%). Short segment stenoses were treated successfully with endoscopic dilation. Mean number of dilations was 1.6 and the mean time from surgery to the initial endoscopic intervention was 48 days. Those with long segment stenoses underwent multiple endoscopic dilation procedures, however ultimately required conversion to RYGB [72]. There is inconsistent and weak data for management of strictures after LSG. The International Sleeve Gastrectomy Expert Panel recommends observation, followed by endoscopic dilation, and reoperation in patients who failed treatment in 6 weeks [73].

Gastric Band

Band Slippage

Gastric band slippage is defined as the prolapse of the gastric wall proximally through the band, and is usually classified as either posterior (upwards herniation of the posterior stomach) or anterior (cephalic prolapse of the stomach's inferior portion) [74,75]. The reported rates of band slippage range from 0% to 24% [75]. Accounting for some of the variability in incidence is the change in operative technique over the years. Posterior slippage is mostly seen in patients with the band placed in a perigastric technique, which requires opening of the lesser sac, as compared to the pars flaccida technique, which leaves the lesser sac intact [75]. A randomized controlled trial between the two techniques reported by O'brien, found the pars flaccida technique resulted in a decreased slip rate compared to the perigastric technique (4% vs 16%). There were no cases of posterior slippage using the pars flaccida technique [76]. Singhal reported a 0.26% rate of slippage with their surgical technique involving gastropexy and gastro-gastro sutures to fix the band [77]. Patients will typically present with epigastric pain, dysphagia, dyspepsia, nausea, and vomiting [78]. Diagnosis is confirmed with abdominal plain radiograph (AXR), computed tomographic scan (CT), or an UGI series. There is an eccentric pouch, with the band in the vertical (posterior slippage) or horizontal (anterior slippage) plane [75]. Consequences of gastric band slippage include obstruction, erosion, ischemia, and perforation of the stomach. Patients with band slippage require deflation of the band. Operative intervention is necessary to reposition the band, or in the case of sepsis or perforation, remove the band.

Band Erosion

Erosion of the band through the stomach wall is a serious complication, reportedly occurring in 1-3% of cases [78,79]. Brown reported a 2.85% incidence from a large prospective database, with 6.8% in the perigastric approach and 1.1% in the pars flaccida approach[79]. Singhal's meta-analysis found a significant correlation between erosion and slippage rates, citing improved surgical technique and band design as a contributing factor to decreased rates over time [77]. Presentation is variable but patients typically describe loss of satiety, abdominal pain, and port swelling [79]. Port-site infection in a patient with a laparoscopic adjustable gastric band is generally considered to be band erosion until proven otherwise. In Brown's series, diagnosis was made definitively by endoscopy. Treatment involved removal of the band, and subsequent replacement at a later time or conversion to a sleeve gastrectomy or bypass [79].

Failure and Revisional Surgery

The effectiveness of bariatric surgery can be assessed by the percentage of excess weight loss (% EWL), as well as by the need for revisional surgery [80]. Analyzing these long-term outcome data is difficult as patients are often lost to follow-up and the reason for reoperation is not always identified. O'brien reported prospective long-term outcomes of LAGB, and found 47% EWL maintained at 15 years. The need for revisional surgery has decreased over time, however nearly 50% of patients underwent a second procedure [81].

Additionally, weight loss in patients who underwent revisional procedures was not significantly different from those who only had one procedure, indicating revision with replacement of the band and conversion to another procedure does not compromise weight loss status. The most common reason to undergo revisional surgery after LAGB is insufficient weight loss. Coblijn concluded that revision to LRGYB or LSG is a feasible option with short-term and long-term complication rates of 8.5 and 15.7%, and 8.9 and 2.5%, respectively [82].

O'brien further performed a systematic review in which the median weight loss was comparable in LAGB and RYGB (54.2% EWL vs 54% EWL), as well as the need for revisional surgery (26% vs 22%) [81]. Nguyen performed a randomized trial between LRYGB and LAGB, and defined treatment failure as the need for conversion to another procedure due to failure of weight loss or <20% EWL, at one year postoperatively the treatment failure rate was 0% and 16.7% for LRYGB and LAGB groups, respectively. When the patients who were lost to follow up were included in the analysis, the treatment failure rate was 15.3% for LRYGB and 23.3% for LAGB [83].

LSG has much less long-term data since it has become a popular procedure only in the last few years. However, a randomized study of 80 patients by Himpens compared LAGB and LSG and found median % EWL at 3 years to be 48% and 66%, respectively. Two patients in the LAGB underwent conversion to LRYGB and two patients in the LSG underwent conversion to duodenal switch, due to weight loss failure [84].

Conclusion

Bariatric surgery has been established as the most successful management of obese patients in a subgroup of the population. The developments of laparoscopy, improved surgical techniques, and evidence-based surgery have resulted in a consistently low mortality and lower complication rates. The complication profile is often unique to the procedures, such as anastomotic leak, stricture, marginal ulcer, internal hernia, vitamin deficiencies, band slippage, and band erosion. While outcomes have improved, the consequences of these events are potentially devastating. A high index of suspicion and low threshold for intervention is paramount in management practices. It is reasonable to expect some bariatric patients to undergo more than one surgical procedure in their lifetime, and still achieve meaningful weight loss.

References

[1]   Ogden, CL; et al. Prevalence of obesity among adults: United States, 2011-2012. *NCHS Data Brief*, 2013 (131), 1-8.

[2]   Gastrointestinal surgery for severe obesity. *Proceedings of a National Institutes of Health Consensus Development Conference*. March 25-27, 1991, Bethesda, MD. *Am J Clin Nutr*, 1992, 55(2 Suppl), 487S-619S.

[3]   Buchwald, H; et al. Metabolic/Bariatric surgery worldwide 2011. *Obes Surg*, 2013, 23, 427-436.

[4]   Karamanakos, SN; et al. Weight loss, appetite suppression, and changes in fasting and postprandial ghrelin and peptide-YY levels after roux-en-y gastric bypass and sleeve gastrectomy: a prospective, double blind study. *Ann Surg*, 2008, 247(3), 401-407.

[5]   Helmio, M; et al. SLEEVEPASS: a randomized prospective multicenter study comparing laparoscopic sleeve gastrectomy and gastric bypass in the treatment of morbid obesity: preliminary results. *Surg endosc*, 2012, 26, 2521-26.

[6]   Tichansky, DS; et al. Operations for morbid obesity. Yeo, CJ, *Shackelford's surgery of the alimentary tract*, 7th ed. Philadelphia, PA: Saunders Elsevier, 2013, 791-802.

[7]   Regan, JP; et al. Early experience with two-stage laparoscopic roux-en-y gastric bypass as an alternative in the super-super obese patient. *Obes Surg*, 2003, 13(6), 861-864.

[8]   Helgstrand, F; et al. Nationwide prospective study of outcomes after elective incisional hernia repair. *J Am Coll Surg*, 2012, 216(2), 217-228.

[9]   Kwaan, MR; et al. Are right-sided colectomy outcomes different from left-sided outcomes?: study of patients with colon cancer in the ACS NSQIP database. *JAMA Surg*, 2013, 148(6), 504-10.

[10] Morino, M; et al. Mortality after bariatric surgery, analysis of 13,871 morbidly obese patients from a national registry. *Ann Surg*, 2007, 246, 1002–1009.

[11] Flum, DR; et al. Perioperative safety in the longitudinal assessment of bariatric surgery. *NEJM*, 2009, 361(5), 445-454.

[12] Hutter, M; et al. First report from the American College of Surgeons Bariatric Surgery Center Network: laparoscopic sleeve gastrectomy has morbidity and effectiveness posititioned between the band and the bypass. *Ann Surg*, 2011, 254(3), 410-20.

[13] Shabanzadeh, DM; et al. Laparoscopic surgery compared with open surgery decreases surgical site infection in obese patients: a systematic review and meta-analysis. *Ann Surg*, 2012, 256(6), 934-945.

[14] Nugyen, NT; et al. Laparoscopic versus open gastric bypass: a randomized study of outcomes, quality of life, and costs. *Ann Surg*, 2001, 234(3), 279-291.

[15] Winegar, DA; et al. Venous thromboembolism after bariatric surgery performed by Bariatric Surgery Center of Excellence Participants: analysis of the Bariatric Outcomes Longitudinal Database. *Surg Obes Relat Dis*, 2011, 7(2), 181-8.

[16] Stein, PD; et al. Pulmonary embolism and deep venous thrombosis following bariatric surgery. *Obes Surg*, 2013, 23, 663–668.

[17] Gould, MK; Garcia, DA; Wren, SM; et al. Prevention of VTE in nonorthopedic surgical patients: antithrombotic therapy and prevention of thrombosis, 9th ed: American College of Chest Physicians evidence-based clinical practice guidelines. *Chest*, 2012, 141(2)(suppl): e227S-e277S.

[18] Silecchia, G; et al. Effectiveness of laparoscopic sleeve gastrectomy (first stage of biliopancreatic diversion with duodenal switch) on comorbidities in super-obese high risk patients. *Obes Surg*, 2006, 16, 1138-44.

[19] Mittermair, R; et al. Results and complications after laparoscopic sleeve gastrectomy. *Surg Today*, 2013, DOI 10.1007/s00595-013-0688-0.

[20] Nguyen, NT; et al. Gastrointestinal hemorrhage after laparoscopic gastric bypass. *Obes Surg*, 2004, 14, 1308-12.

[21] Harakeh, AB. Complications of laparoscopic roux-en-y gastric bypass. *Surg Clin North Am*, 2011, 91(6), 1225-1237.

[22] Fernandez, AZ; Jr. DeMaria, EJ; Tichansky, DS; et al. Experience with over 3,000 open and laparoscopic bariatric procedures: multivariate analysis of factors related to leak and resultant mortality. *Surg Endosc*, 2004, 18(2), 193–7.

[23] Fox, SR; et al. Leaks and gastric disruption in bariatric surgery. Buchwald H, et al. *Surgical Management of Obesity*, 1st ed. Philadelphia, PA: Saunders Elsevier, 2007, 304-312.

[24] Ballesta, C; Berindoague, R; Cabrera, M; et al. Management of anastomotic leaks after laparoscopic roux-en-y gastric bypass. *Obes Surg*, 2008, 18(6), 623–30.

[25] Da Costa, M; Mata, A; Espinos, J; et al. Endoscopic dilation of gastrojejunal anastomotic strictures after laparoscopic gastric bypass. Predictors of initial failure. *Obes Surg*, 2011, (1), 36–41.

[26] Goitein, D; Papasavas, PK; Gagne, D; et al. Gastrojejunal strictures following laparoscopic Roux-en-Y gastric bypass for morbid obesity. *Surg Endosc*, 2005, 19, 628–32.

[27] Go, MR; Muscarella, II P; Needleman, BJ; et al. Endoscopic management of stomal stenosis after Roux-en-Y gastric bypass. *Surg Endosc*, 2004, 18, 56–9.

[28] Ukleja, A; Afonso, BB; Pimentel, R; et al. Outcome of endoscopic balloon dilation of strictures after laparoscopic gastric bypass. *Surg Endosc*, 2008, 22, 1746–50.

[29] Nguyen, NT; Stevens, CM; Wolfe, BM. Incidence and outcome of anastomotic stricture after laparoscopic gastric bypass. *J Gastrointest Sug*, 2003, 7, 997–1003.

[30] Rossi, TR; Dynda, D; Estes, NC; et al. Stricture dilation after laparoscopic Roux-en-Y gastric bypass. *Am J Surg*, 2005, 189, 357–60.

[31] Gould, JC; Garren, M; Boll, V; et al. The impact of circular stapler diameter on the incidence of gastrojejunostomy stenosis and weight loss following laparoscopic Roux-en-Y gastric bypass. *Surg Endosc*, 2006, 20, 1017–20.

[32] Rasmussen, JJ; et al. Marginal ulceration after laparoscopic gastric bypass: an analysis of predisposing factors in 260 patients. *Surg endosc*, 2007, (7), 1090-4.

[33] Dallal, RM; et al. Ulcer disease after gastric bypass surgery. *Surg Obes Rel Dis*, 2006, 2(4), 455-9.

[34] Gumbs, AA; et al. Incidence and management of marginal ulceration after laparoscopic Roux-Y gastric bypass. *Surg Obes Relat Dis.*, 2006, 2(4), 460-3.

[35] Azagury, DE; et al. Marginal ulceration after Roux-en-Y gastric bypass surgery: characteristics, risk factors, treatment, and outcomes. Endosc, 2011, 43(11), 950-4.

[36] Arts, J; et al. Efficacy of the long-acting repeatable formulation of the somatostatin analogue octreotide in postoperative dumping. *Clinical gastr and hepatology*, 2009, 7, 432-437.

[37] Mallory, GN; Macgregor, AM; Rand, CS. The influence of dumping on weight loss after gastric restrictive surgery for morbid obesity. *Obes Surg*, 1996, 6, 474–478.

[38] Cawley, J; et al. Predicting complications after bariatric surgery using obesity-related co-morbidities. *Obes Surg*, 2007, 17, 1451-56.

[39] Banerjee, A; et al. The role of dumping syndrome in weight loss after gastric bypass surgery. *Surg endosc*, 2013, 27(5), 1573-8.

[40] Podnos, YD; Jimenez, JC; Wilson, SE; Stevens, CM; Nguyen, NT. Complications after laparoscopic gastric bypass: a review of 3464 cases. *Arch Surg*, 2003, 138, 957–961.

[41] Nguyen, N; Huerta, S; Gelfand, D; Stevens, M; Jeffrey, J. Bowel obstruction after laparoscopic Roux-en-Y gastric bypass. *Obes Surg*, 2004, 14, 190–196.

[42] Husain, S; Ahmed, A; Johnson, J; Boss, T; O'Malley, W. Small bowel obstruction after laparoscopic Roux-en-Y gastric bypass. *Arch Surg*, 2007, 142, 988–993.

[43] Koppman, JS; Li, C; Gandas, A. Small bowel obstruction after laparoscopic Roux-en-Y gastric bypass: A review of 9,527 patients. *J Am Coll Surg*, 2008, 206, 571–584.

[44] Obeid, A; et al. Internal hernia after laparoscopic roux-en-Y gastric bypass. *J gastrointes surg*, 2013. DOI 10.1007/s11605-013-2377-0.

[45] Iannelli, A; et al. Internal hernia after laparoscopic roux-en-Y gastric bypass for morbid obesity. *Obesity Surg*, 2006, 16, 1265-1271.

[46] Steele, KE; Prokopowicz, GP; Magnuson, T; Lidor, A; Schweitzer, M. Laparoscopic antecolic Roux-en-Y gastric bypass with closure of internal defects leads to fewer internal hernias than the retrocolic approach. *Surg Endosc*, 2008, 22, 2056–2061.

[47] Alvarez-Leite, JI. Nutrient deficiencies secondary to bariatric surgery. *Curr Opin Clin Nutr Metab Care*, 2004, 7, 569–75.

[48] Vargas-Ruiz, AG; Hernandez-Rivera, G; Herrera, MF. Prevalence of iron, folate, and vitamin B12 defciency anemia after laparoscopic Roux-en-Y gastric bypass. *Obes Surg*, 2008, 18, 288–93.

[49] Shankar, P; et al. Micronutrient deficiencies after bariatric surgery. *Nutrition*, 2010, 26, 1031-1037.

[50] Brolin, RE; Leung, M. Survey of vitamin and mineral supplementation after gastric bypass and biliopancreatic diversion for morbid obesity. *Obes Surg*, 1999, 9, 150-154.

[51] Brolin, RE; LaMarca, LB; Kenler, HA; et al. Malabsorptive gastric bypass in patients with superobesity. *J Gastrointest Surg*, 2002, 6, 195-203, discussion 4-5.

[52] Bloomberg, RD; et al. Nutritional deficiencies following bariatric surgery: what have we learned? *Obes Surg*, 2005, 5(2), 145-54.

[53] Lakhani, SV; Shah, HN; Alexander, K; Finelle, FC; Kirkpatrick, JR; Koch, TR. Small intestinal bacterial overgrowth and thiamin deficiency after Roux-en-Y gastric bypass surgery in obese patients. *Nutr Res*, 2008, 28, 293–8.

[54] Aasheim, ET. Wernicke encephalopathy after bariatric surgery - A systematic review. *Ann Surg*, 2008, 248, 714–20.

[55] Clements, RH; Yellumahanthi, K; Wesley, M; Ballem, N; Bland, KI. Hyperparathyroidism and vitamin D defciency after laparoscopic gastric bypass. *Am Surg*, 2008, 74, 469–74.

[56] Coates, PS; Fernstrom, JD; Fernstrom, MH; et al. Gastric bypass surgery for morbid obesity leads to an increase in bone turnover and a decrease in bone mass. *J Clin Endocrinol Metab*, 2004, 89, 1061-1065.

[57] Clements, RH; Katasani, VG; Palepu, R; Leeth, RR; Leath, TD; Roy, BP; et al. Incidence of vitamin deficiency after laparoscopic Roux-en-Y gastric bypass in a university hospital setting. *Am Surg*, 2006, 72, 1196–204.

[58] Lee, WB; Hamilton, SM; Harris, JP; Schwab, IR. Ocular complications of hypovitaminosis after bariatric surgery. *Ophthalmology*, 2005, 112, 1031–4.

[59] Diniz, M de F; Diniz, MT; Sanches, SR; Salgado, PP; Valada~o, MM; Arau´ jo, FC; et al. Elevated serum parathormone after Roux-en-Y gastric bypass. *Obes Surg*, 2004, 14, 1222–6.

[60] Lalor, PF; Tucker, ON; Szomstein, S; et al. Complications after laparoscopic sleeve gastrectomy. *Surg Obes Relat Dis*, 2008, 4(1), 33–8.

[61] Casella, G; et al. Nonsurgical treatment of staple line leaks after laparoscopic sleeve gastrectomy. *Obes Surg*, 2009 (7), 821-6.

[62] Aurora, AR; et al. Sleeve gastrectomy and the risk of leak: a systematic analysis of 4,888 patients. *Surg endosc*, 2012, 26, 1509-15.

[63] Parikh, M; et al. Surgical strategies that may decrease leak after laparoscopic sleeve gastrectomy: as systematic review and meta-analysis of 9991 cases. *Ann Surg*, 2013, 257(2), 231-237.

[64] Knapps, J; Ghanem, M; Clements, J; Merchant, AM. A systematic review of staple-line reinforcement in laparoscopic sleeve gastrectomy. *JSLS*, 2013, 17(3), 390-9.

[65] Sanchez-Santos, R; Masdevall, C; Baltasar, A; et al. Short- and mid-term outcomes of sleeve gastrectomy for morbid obesity: the experience of the Spanish National Registry. *Obes Surg*, 2009, 19, 1203–1210.

[66] Soricelli, E; Casella, G; Rizzello, M; et al. Initial experience with laparoscopic crural closure in the management of hiatal hernia in obese

patients undergoing sleeve gastrectomy. *Obes Surg*, 2010, 20(8), 1149–53.

[67] Hamoui, N; Anthone, GJ; Kaufman, HS; et al. Sleeve gastrectomy in the high-risk patient. *Obes Surg*, 2006, 16(11), 1445–9.

[68] Nocca, D; Krawczykowsky, D; Bomans, B; et al. A prospective multicenter study of 163 sleeve gastrectomies: results at 1 and 2 years. *Obes Surg*, 2008, 18(5), 560–5.

[69] Himpens, J; et al. Long-term results of laparoscopic sleeve gastrectomy for obesity. *Ann Surg*, 2010, 252(2), 319-24.

[70] Daes, J; et al. Laparoscopic sleeve gastrectomy: symptoms of gastroesophageal reflux can be reduced by changes in surgical technique. *Obes Surg*, 2012, (12), 1874-9.

[71] Shnell, M; et al. Balloon dilation for symptomatic gastric sleeve stricture. *Gast endosc*, 2013. DOI: 10.1016/j.gie2013.09.026.

[72] Parikh, A; et al. Management options for symptomatic stenosis after laparoscopic vertical sleeve gastrectomy in the morbidly obese. *Surg Endosoc*, 2012, 26(3), 738-46.

[73] Burgos, AM; Csendes, A; Braghetto, I. Gastric stenosis after laparoscopic sleeve gastrectomy in morbidly obese patients. *Obes Surg*, 2013, 23, 1481–1486.

[74] Singhal, R; Bryant, C; Kitchen, M; Khan, KS; Deeks, J; Guo, B; Super, P. Band slippage and erosion after laparoscopic gastric banding: a meta-analysis. *Surg Endosc.*, 2010, 12, 2980-6.

[75] Egan, RJ; Monkhouse, SJ; Meredith, HE; Bates, SE; Morgan, JD; Norton, SA. The reporting of gastric band slip and related complications; a review of the literature. *Obes Surg*, 2011, (8), 1280-8.

[76] O'Brien, P; Dixon, J; Laurie, C; et al. A prospective randomised trial of placement of the laparoscopic adjustable gastric band: comparison of the perigastric and pars flaccida pathways. *Obes Surg*, 2005, 15, 820–6.

[77] Singhal, R; Kitchen, M; Ndirika, S; Hunt, K; Bridgwater, S; Super, P. The "Birmingham stitch": avoiding slippage in laparoscopic gastric banding. *Obes Surg*, 2008, 18, 359–363.

[78] Owers, C; Ackroyd, R. A study examining the complications associated with gastric banding. *Obes Surg*, 2013, 1, 56-9.

[79] Brown, WA; Egberts, KJ; Franke-Richard, D; Thodiyil, P; Anderson, ML; O'Brien, PE. Erosions after laparoscopic adjustable gastric banding: diagnosis and management. *Ann Surg*, 2013, 257(6), 1047-52.

[80] Valezi, AC; et al. Weight Loss Outcome After Roux-en-Y Gastric Bypass: 10 Years of Follow-up. *Obes surg*, 2013, 23, 1290-93.

[81] O'Brien, PE; MacDonald, L; Anderson, M; Brennan, L; Brown, WA. Long-term outcomes after bariatric surgery: fifteen-year follow-up of adjustable gastric banding and a systematic review of the bariatric surgical literature. *Ann Surg*, 2013, 257(1), 87-94.

[82] Coblijn, UK; Verveld, CJ; van Wagensveld, BA; Lagarde, SM. Laparoscopic Roux-en-Y gastric bypass or laparoscopic sleeve gastrectomy as revisional procedure after adjustable gastric band--a systematic review. *Obes Surg*, 2013, 23(11), 1899-914.

[83] Nguyen, NT; Slone, JA; Nguyen, XM; Hartman, JS; Hoyt, DB. A prospective randomized trial of laparoscopic gastric bypass versus laparoscopic adjustable gastric banding for the treatment of morbid obesity: outcomes, quality of life, and costs. *Ann Surg*, 2009, 250(4), 631-41.

[84] Himpens, J; et al. A prospective randomized study between laparoscopic gastric banding and laparoscopic isolated sleeve gastrectomy: results after 1 and 3 years. *Obes Surg*, 2006, 16(11), 1450-6.

In: General and Abdominal Surgery
Editor: Kassandra Sarah Slavomir

ISBN: 978-1-63117-440-7
© 2014 Nova Science Publishers, Inc.

Chapter 3

Atrial Fibrillation after Surgery

***Di Ai, MD, PhD and Juan P. Cata, MD**[*]*
Department of Anesthesiology and Perioperative Medicine,
University of Texas -MD Anderson Cancer Center,
Houston, Texas - US

Abstract

Postoperative atrial fibrillation is a common supraventricular arrhythmia in the context of thoracic cardiac and non-cardiac surgery. In contrast, the incidence of this arrhythmia is very low after non-thoracic non-cardiac surgery. Common risks factor include age, male gender, history of atrial fibrillation, coronary artery disease and atrial enlargement. Inflammation, oxidative stress and surgery-induced release of catecholamines have been implicated in the physiopathology of postoperative atrial fibrillation; hence, several pharmacological interventions have been tried to reduce its incidence. To date, betablockers and amiodarone have shown the most promising benefits in terms of prophylaxis.

[*] Corresponding author: Juan P. Cata, MD, Department of Anesthesiology and Perioperative Medicine, Unit 0408 The University of Texas MD Anderson Cancer Center , 1515 Holcombe Boulevard, Houston, TX 77030 USA, Email: jcata@mdanderson.org, Telephone: 713-792-4582, Fax: 713-745-2956

Keywords: Atrial fibrillation, arrhythmia, postoperative, cardiac surgery, noncardiac surgery

Introduction

Atrial fibrillation (AF) is one of the most common cardiac arrhythmia in the general population. Its prevalence is between 0.4% and 1%and has increased in the past 20 years due to the growing aging population (4.6% in > 65 years; 8% in people older than 80), the rising prevalence of chronic heart disease, more frequent diagnosis and better diagnostic techniques [1, 2].

Postoperative cardiac arrhythmias are being increasingly recognized and becoming a major source of morbidity after cardiac and non-cardiac surgery [3, 4]. The incidence of any arrhythmia postoperatively can be up to 85% and their clinical consequences range from transient hypoxemia, cardiac ischemia, hemodynamic instability and perioperative stroke [5, 6]. Postoperative atrial fibrillation (POAF) is the most common serious arrhythmia that occurs during postoperative hospitalization [7]. The incidence of POAF has been documented as up to 60% and 20% after cardiac and noncardiac surgery, respectively [8-11]. Atrial fibrillation after cardiac surgery has been well studied and is associated with a prolonged recovery time, increased morbidity, longer hospital stay and higher health care costs [8].

This chapter will focus on the current knowledge of POAF in the following aspects, including incidence, risk factors, mechanisms and prophylaxis in both cardiac surgery and noncardiac surgery.

Postoperative Atrial Fibrillation After Cardiac Surgery

The incidence of POAF after cardiac surgery ranges from 10% to 60% [8-10]. Several reasons can explain this wide range of incidences. For instance, the definition of POAF varies from study to study. Some studies defined POAF as an episode lasting longer than 5 minutes, while other studies only included those that lasted longer than 10 minutes [12, 13]. Race and ethnicity has been shown to influence the incidence of POAF. Thus, it has been reported a similar incidence in USA (33.7%) and Europe (34%), but lower in Asia (15.7%) and Africa (17.4%) [8]. The incidence also depends on the type of cardiac surgery. For example, the incidence of this arrhythmia after coronary artery bypass grafting (CABG) surgery ranges from 16 to 50%, [14-17] and appears to be higher after valve surgery and the highest after the combination of CABG and valve surgery [13, 16, 18, 19]. Interestingly, the incidence of POAF is very low in heart transplantation cases (4%), which may be due to the significantly reduced atrial size and isolated pulmonary veins of the transplanted heart [20].

The duration of the postoperative monitoring is another factor why clinical studies have reported different incidences of POAF. Shen et al. reported an incidence of 29% when patients were monitored during their whole stay in hospital; [17] in contrast, Silbert et al. observed a much lower incidence (17.2%) in patients who were only electrocardiographically monitored in the first 48 hours after surgery [16]. Seventy percent of POAF after cardiac surgery have been reported to occur in the first 4 days after surgery, and only 6% of them occurred after the 6th day [12, 20, 21].

Table 1. Risk factors of AF

POAF cardiac surgery	POAF non-cardiac surgery

• **Acute**
Direct cardiac irritation
• **Chronic**
Advanced age
Structural heart disease
  Left atrial enlargement
  Mitral valve disease
  Congestive heart failure
  Hypertension
History of atrial fibrillation
Prior myocardial infarction
Myocardial ischemia
Male sex
Pulmonary disease
  Chronic Obstructive Lung Disease
Preoperative digoxin use
Hypoxia
Hypovolemia
Electrolyte abnormalities:
  Hypokalemia
  Hypomagnesemia
Hypothyroidism
	• Advanced age
	• Male gender
	• Types of pulmonary resection
	• Structural heart disease:
	• Congestive heart failure
	• History of hypertension
	• Cardiac enlargement
	• History of atrial fibrillation
	• Ischemic changes on ECG
	• Prior myocardial infarction

The table shows the proposed risk factors involved in the physiopathogenesis.
POAF after thoracic cardiac and non-cardiac surgery.

Postoperative atrial fibrillation after cardiac surgery is multi-factorial. Its predisposing factors can be classified as acute, such as direct surgical intervention and chronic, such as aging and structural heart disease [9] (Table 1). Advanced age is an independent chronic risk factor for the occurrence of new onset of AF, not only because of the known changes that the myocardium undergo while aging (atrial fibrosis and loss of atrial muscle mass), but also the increased incidence of coronary artery disease [1, 22, 23]. Structural heart disease, such as left atrial enlargement, mitral valve disease, congestive heart failure, and hypertension are well known risk factors of non-surgery AF [24] and are also associated with POAF [20, 25]. A canine model showed that chronic left atrial dilatation due to mitral regurgitation increased the vulnerability to AF; interestingly, chronic inflammation and increased interstitial fibrosis was revealed in the atria of the animals that developed the arrhythmia [26]. Chronic heart failure can cause left atrial dilatation by increasing atrial filling pressures and ensued atrial fibrosis [27, 28]. Systemic elevated blood pressure causes left ventricular hypertrophy, left atrial dilatation but unfortunately, angiotensin-converting enzyme inhibitor (ACE-I) or angiotensin receptor blocker has not been shown to decrease the incidence of POAF [1, 29, 30].

Inflammation has been shown to play a prominent role in the development of POAF after cardiac surgery [9]. During cardiopulmonary bypass surgery, activation of the complement cascade and release of inflammatory cytokines have been implicated in the genesis of atrial fibrillation [31-33]. For instance, the C-reactive protein concentration curve is consistent with the onset curve of POAF [9]. Furthermore, Fontes et al., reported that perioperative activation of monocytes and higher circulating monocyte and neutrophils were associated with POAF [34]. Local surgical trauma and even mild atrial inflammation due to pericardiotomy also contribute in the pathogenesis of POAF. Frustaci et al. reported lymphomono nuclear infiltrates in atrial tissue of 66% of patients [35]. Similarly, Chen et al. observed a significantly high amount of CD45 (+) cells in right atrial appendages of AF patients. [36] Interestingly, in a canine sterile of pericardit is model the development of AF was inhibited by the administration of steroids and statins [37]. In line with these observations, clinical trials that administered steroids have also shown to reduce the incidence of POAF by inhibition of cytokine release, such as tumor necrosis factor α and IL-6 [38]. Preoperative statin use was associated with a 34% reduction in the risk of new-onset atrial fibrillation after surgery. The mechanisms by which statins might help reduce the POAF include lowering inflammation markers [39] and attenuating myocardial reperfusion [40].

Sympathetic stimulation is another facilitating trigger for development of AF after cardiac surgery because of the excitatory effects of catecholamines on the excitability and automaticity on the cardiac pacemaker cells [41]. Kalman et al. showed that the concentrations of norepinephrine in the right atria were elevated in post CABG surgery patients, suggesting that pathogenesis of POAF might be mediated by sympathetic activation [41, 42]. Elevated norepinephrine concentrations were detected in advanced age population as well [43]. An increase of heart rate variability prior to POAF was reported in patients who developed POAF, consistent with sympathetic activation [44, 45]. Interestingly, although the peak of sympathetic activation occurs within 24 hours postoperatively, and most of POAFs develop during 48 and 72 hours, successful blocking of the beta-adrenoceptors has been used successfully in the prophylaxis of AF after cardiac surgery [46].

Oxidative stress is another acute mechanism that contributes to POAF after cardiac surgery. After reperfusion, the production of reactive oxygen species increases and this might result in myocardial damage and cell death [47, 48]. Antioxidant drugs, such as ascorbic acid and N-acetylcysteine, might lower the incidence of POAF after CABG surgery; more interestingly, the combination of ascorbic acid and beta-blockers seems to be more effective than beta-blockade alone [49-51]. In addition, statins may also decrease the incidence of POAF due to their known antioxidative properties [52].

Although functional changes in L- type Ca^{2+} channel have been implicated in shortening of atrial refractoriness and AF, Workman et al. could not find out any differences in L- type Calcium channel between patients with or without POAF [53-55]. Preexistent structural alterations such as atrial remodeling caused by aging, [56] increased amount of fibrosis in right atrial appendages, [57] and left atrial enlargement can predispose to POAF [58]. Specifically, connexin 40 builds up transmembrane channels in atrial myocytes and higher connexin 40 expression has been associated with the chronic change observed in patients who developed POAF [59].

Many drugs, including beta-blocker, amiodarone, sotalol, calcium channel blockers (CCB) and statins, have been investigated in the prophylaxis of POAF (Table 2). Beta-blockers can decrease sympathetic tone and lower the incidence of dysrhythmias. From 1979 to 2001, 29 trials were conducted to test betra-blocker perioperatively. Thirteen of them showed prophylaxis with significant reduction of AF after surgery [60-64]. The combination of beta-blockers plus digitalis has also been studied in the prophylaxis of POAF [65, 66]. Sotalol is an anti-arrhythmic drug that has both beta-blocker and potassium blocker properties. Sotalol has shown to lower the incidence of AF by 41% to 93% comparing with placebo [67-72]. This anti-arrhythmic is usually well tolerated; however, it is recommended the monitoring of the QT interval during its administration and careful titration in patients with renal insufficiency. Few studies, with conflicting results, have compared the efficacy of sotalol and beta-blockers [63, 73, 74].

Amiodarone is a commonly used anti-arrhythmic drug that has multiple ion channels and beta-blocker properties. Trials assessing the efficacy of amiodarone had showed 8% to 72% relative reduction in the incidence of POAF [75-83]. Side effects such as bradycardia have been reported but uncommon [75, 79, 80, 82]. It is unclear whether amiodarone is a better prophylaxis than beta-blockers for POAF after cardiac surgery, although a study showed a trend favoring amiodarone [78, 84].

The success of nondihydropyridine CCB, like diltiazem and verapamil, in the prevention of POAF is limited and with mixed results [85-88]. Digitalis is another anti-arrhythmic drug that increases the vagal tone and reduces the ventricular rate during AF. Unfortunately, the results from studies that have evaluated the efficacy of digitalis in the context of POAF are dismal [64, 66, 89-94]. Depletion of intracellular magnesium can predispose patients to postoperative arrhythmias [95]. Although magnesium sulfate treatment does not result in prophylaxis against POAF, serum magnesium should be monitored and maintained in those patients who undergoing cardiac surgery [60, 64, 95, 96].

Postoperative Atrial Fibrillation After Non-Cardiac Surgery

Atrial fibrillation is also a common arrhythmia after thoracic non-cardiac surgery; it incidence ranges from 5% to 20% depending on the type of surgery performed [7, 11, 17, 97, 98]. For instance, the incidence after lung lobectomy ranges between 12% to 30% and 23% to 67% after pneumonectomy [25, 99-103]. In agreement with the literature, data from our group indicate that 19.4% of the patients develop AF after lung cancer surgery (unpublished data). Esophagectomies are also common non-cardiac thoracic surgeries. The incidence of postesophagectomy AF is between 13% and 46% [99, 104, 105]. Data from our group show that 12.7% of the patients who underwent esophagectomy developed AF (unpublished data). The average time of onset of POAF after non-cardiac surgery is 2-3 days [106]. In our center, 50.7% and 47.4% of the patients developed AF in the first 48 hours after lung and esophageal surgery, respectively (unpublished data).

The incidence of AF after non-cardiac, non-thoracic surgery is much lower than that after thoracic surgery. Sohn et al. reported a very low incidence of AF 0.39% in a group of patients who underwent non-cardiac non-thoracic surgery [107]. Christians et al. reported similar low incidence of AF (0.37%) and identified preexisting cardiovascular risk factors such as hypertension, prior history of atrial fibrillation, valvular disease or myocardial infarction to be associated the development of POAF [108].

The risk factors that have been associated with POAF after noncardiac surgery are similar to those involved in POAF after cardiac surgery [99]. Passman et al. identified male gender as independent risk factor [25]. African-American race was associated with a lower risk of POAF, which is consistent with the findings in cardiac surgery [109]. Vaporciyan et al. reported that advanced age was an independent risk factor in their 2588 patients study: age 50 to 59 years (RR: 1.70, 95% CI = 1.01- 2.88); age 60 to 69 years (RR: 4.49, 95% CI = 2.79- 7.22); age >70 years (RR: 5.30, 95% CI = 3.28- 8.59). The type of intrathoracic surgery appears to be significant risk factor for the development of POAF; for instance, mediastinal tumor resection (RR: 2.36, 95% CI = 0.95 – 5.88), lobectomy (RR: 3.89, 95% CI = 2.19- 6.91), bilobectomy (RR: 7.16, 95% CI = 3.02- 16.96), pneumonectomy (RR: 8.91, 95% CI = 4.59- 17.28) and esophagectomy (RR: 2.95, 95% CI = 1.55- 5.62) are all independent predictors of POAF [99]. Roselli et al. reported heart failure and history of AF as independent risk factors [110]. Interestingly, elevated preoperative plasma concentrations of atrial natriuretic peptide, B-type natriuretic peptide and N-terminal BNP were also associated with the development of AF. [111] In this regard, increased left or right heart pressure might be a potential mechanism of POAF after pulmonary resection. Amar et al. reported that increased right heart pressures but not fluid overload or right heart enlargement predisposes to clinically significant SVT after pulmonary resection. Importantly, the authors found that an increased tricuspid regurgitation jet velocity was an independent risk factor for POAF [112].

Comparing to studies addressing the issue of AF after cardiac surgery, less data exist regarding mechanisms of AF after non-cardiac surgery [9, 106]. The effect of inflammation on post-pulmonary resection is controversial. Amar et al., did not find that the plasma concentrations of inflammatory markers (IL-6 and CRP) in POAF patients were associated with the onset of POAF, although, in the same study statins which have anti-inflammatory properties did lower the incidence of POAF [113].

Table 2. Proposed mechanisms of POAF and prophylactic interventions

- **Inflammation**
  Steroids
  Statins

- **Sympathetic activation**
  Beta-blockers
  Calcium channel blockers
  Amiodarone
  Sotalol

- **Oxidative stress**
  Statins
  Antioxidants

- **Ion channel alterations**
  Calcium channel blockers
  Amiodarone
  Sotalol

Beta-blockers, calcium channel blockers and amiodarone have been broadly evaluated as potential prophylactic drugs of POAF after cardiac surgery, but only a few studies were conducted after noncardiac surgery. Jacobsen et al. randomized patients who had lung resection to 100 mg metoprolol or placebo and found that the incidence of AF lasting more than 30 seconds was significantly lower in metoprolol group (6.7%) than in the placebo group (40.0%) [114].

In another randomized, placebo-controlled study in which propranolol was given to patients who underwent lobectomies, pneumonectomy or es-ophagectomies the incidence of postoperative tachyarrhythmias (including supraventricular tachycardia and ventricular tachycardia) that required treatment was 6% in the propranolol group versus 20% in the control group. It is important to mention that in both studies hypotension and bradycardia were significantly higher in the beta-blocker group [114, 115].

Amarand et al. evaluated the efficacy of diltiazem, digoxin and placebo in a group of lung resection patients. Both drugs were given intravenously for the first 36 hours after surgery, and then taken orally for one month. The authors concluded that there were not significantly differences in the incidences of

POAF between the groups [116]. In another study conducted by the same author in which patients were randomized to intra- and postoperative diltiazem versus placebo, the incidence of POAF in the diltiazem group was significant lower than in the placebo group (15% versus 25%) [117]. The effect of verapamil has also been investigated. One study found no difference in the incidence of POAF between verapamil-or placebo-treated patients (8% versus 15%, respectively). Interestingly, those patients treated with verapamil had substantially more episodes of hypotension and bradycardia [118]. To complicate more this matter, Lindgren et al. found that verapamil was associated with a significantly lower incidence POAF [119].

Amiodarone has also been studied in the context of POAF after non-cardiac surgery. In a study conducted by Lanza et al. amiodarone treated patients developed significantly fewer episodes of AF than the control group (9.7% versus 33%, respectively) [120]. Tisdale et al. conducted a prospective controlled unblinded study in which amiodarone was intravenously administered for the first 24 hours postoperatively and then orally for 6 days or until discharge. The incidence of AF that needed treatments was significantly lower in amiodarone-treated patients than in the control group (13.8% versus32.3%, respectively), but the incidence of bradycardia (heart rate lower 50 bpm) was much higher than in the control group (6.2% versus 1.5%, respectively); suggesting ECG monitoring is required in amiodarone treated group [106].

Statins are cholesterol-lowering medications with anti-inflammatory properties. In a study by Amar et al. who included patients who had lobecto-mies or pneumonectomies, the incidence of POAF was significantly lower in statin treatment group than non-statin group (11% versus 29%) [113]. As previously mentioned, electrolyte imbalances in particular hypomagnesemia can trigger POAF. Terzi et al. reported that patients who received intravenous magnesium as a preventive of AF after pneumonectomy or intrapericardial procedure had a lower incidence than control group (10.7% versus 26.7%, respectively) [121].

In conclusion PAOF after cardiothoracic surgery is a common entity associated with increased morbidity, mortality and prolonged hospital stay. [144]. More patients undergoing non-cardiac surgery suffer AF than patients undergoing cardiac surgery since much more non-cardiac surgeries are operated than cardiac surgery a year around the world. Some predisposing risk factors of POAF, like advanced age and history of AF, are shared by both non-cardiac and cardiac surgery. The type of lung resection appears to be a specific risk factor for the development of AF afternoon-cardiac surgery. So far, the only consistent preoperative risk factor for POAF is age (greater than 60 years old). The mechanisms of POAF after non-cardiac surgery are not well known compared to that of AF after cardiac surgery. One potential mechanism of AF post non-cardiac surgery is the increased left or right heart pressure. Inflammation, although being one main mechanism of AF post cardiac surgery, is controversial in that of AF post non-cardiac surgery. Among prophylaxis assessed in clinical trials, beta-blocker and amiodarone have shown to lower the incidence of POAF.

References

[1] Fuster V, Ryden LE, Cannom DS, Crijns HJ, Curtis AB, Ellenbogen KA, Halperin JL, Le Heuzey JY, Kay GN, Lowe JE et al: ACC/AHA/ESC 2006 Guidelines for the Management of Patients with Atrial Fibrillation: a report of the American College of Cardiology/American Heart Association Task Force on Practice Guidelines and the European Society of Cardiology Committee for Practice Guidelines (Writing Committee to Revise the 2001 Guidelines for the Management of Patients With Atrial Fibrillation): developed in collaboration with the European Heart Rhythm Association and the Heart Rhythm Society. *Circulation* 2006, 114(7):e257-354.

[2] Murphy NF, Simpson CR, Jhund PS, Stewart S, Kirkpatrick M, Chalmers J, MacIntyre K, McMurray JJ: A national survey of the prevalence, incidence, primary care burden and treatment of atrial fibrillation in Scotland. *Heart* 2007, 93(5):606-612.

[3] Gajulapalli RD, Rader F: Post Operative Arrhythmias.

[4] Hollenberg SM, Dellinger RP: Noncardiac surgery: postoperative arrhythmias. *Critical care medicine* 2000, 28(10 Suppl):N145-150.

[5] Sloan SB, Weitz HH: Postoperative arrhythmias and conduction disorders. *Med Clin North Am* 2001, 85(5):1171-1189.

[6] Creswell LL: The problem of atrial arrhythmias after noncardiac thoracic surgery. *The Journal of thoracic and cardiovascular surgery* 2004, 127(3):629-630.

[7] Lauer MS, Eagle KA, Buckley MJ, DeSanctis RW: Atrial fibrillation following coronary artery bypass surgery. *Prog Cardiovasc Dis* 1989, 31(5):367-378.

[8] Mathew JP, Fontes ML, Tudor IC, Ramsay J, Duke P, Mazer CD, Barash PG, Hsu PH, Mangano DT, Investigators of the Ischemia R et al:

A multicenter risk index for atrial fibrillation after cardiac surgery. *JAMA: the journal of the American Medical Association* 2004, 291(14):1720-1729.

[9] Maesen B, Nijs J, Maessen J, Allessie M, Schotten U: Post-operative atrial fibrillation: a maze of mechanisms. Europace : European pacing, arrhythmias, and cardiac electrophysiology: *journal of the working groups on cardiac pacing, arrhythmias, and cardiac cellular electrophysiology of the European Society of Cardiology* 2012, 14(2):159-174.

[10] Alqahtani AA: Atrial fibrillation post cardiac surgery trends toward management. *Heart views : the official journal of the Gulf Heart Association* 2010, 11(2):57-63.

[11] Walsh SR, Tang T, Wijewardena C, Yarham SI, Boyle JR, Gaunt ME: Postoperative arrhythmias in general surgical patients. *Annals of the Royal College of Surgeons of England* 2007, 89(2):91-95.

[12] Auer J, Weber T, Berent R, Ng CK, Lamm G, Eber B: Risk factors of postoperative atrial fibrillation after cardiac surgery. *Journal of cardiac surgery* 2005, 20(5):425-431.

[13] Zangrillo A, Landoni G, Sparicio D, Benussi S, Aletti G, Pappalardo F, Fracasso G, Fano G, Crescenzi G: Predictors of atrial fibrillation after off-pump coronary artery bypass graft surgery. *Journal of cardiothoracic and vascular anesthesia* 2004, 18(6):704-708.

[14] Banach M, Rysz J, Drozdz JA, Okonski P, Misztal M, Barylski M, Irzmanski R, Zaslonka J: Risk factors of atrial fibrillation following coronary artery bypass grafting: a preliminary report. *Circulation journal: official journal of the Japanese Circulation Society* 2006, 70(4):438-441.

[15] Ahlsson A, Fengsrud E, Bodin L, Englund A: Postoperative atrial fibrillation in patients undergoing aortocoronary bypass surgery carries an eightfold risk of future atrial fibrillation and a doubled cardiovascular mortality. *European journal of cardio-thoracic surgery: official journal of the European Association for Cardio-thoracic Surgery* 2010, 37(6):1353-1359.

[16] Siebert J, Anisimowicz L, Lango R, Rogowski J, Pawlaczyk R, Brzezinski M, Beta S, Narkiewicz M: Atrial fibrillation after coronary artery bypass grafting: does the type of procedure influence the early postoperative incidence? *European journal of cardio-thoracic surgery: official journal of the European Association for Cardio-thoracic Surgery* 2001, 19(4):455-459.

[17] Shen J, Lall S, Zheng V, Buckley P, Damiano RJ, Jr., Schuessler RB: The persistent problem of new-onset postoperative atrial fibrillation: a single-institution experience over two decades. *The Journal of thoracic and cardiovascular surgery* 2011, 141(2):559-570.

[18] Creswell LL, Schuessler RB, Rosenbloom M, Cox JL: Hazards of postoperative atrial arrhythmias. *The Annals of thoracic surgery* 1993, 56(3):539-549.

[19] Mariscalco G, Engstrom KG: Postoperative atrial fibrillation is associated with late mortality after coronary surgery, but not after valvular surgery. *The Annals of thoracic surgery* 2009, 88(6):1871-1876.

[20] Aranki SF, Shaw DP, Adams DH, Rizzo RJ, Couper GS, VanderVliet M, Collins JJ, Jr., Cohn LH, Burstin HR: Predictors of atrial fibrillation after coronary artery surgery. Current trends and impact on hospital resources. *Circulation* 1996, 94(3):390-397.

[21] Auer J, Weber T, Berent R, Puschmann R, Hartl P, Ng CK, Schwarz C, Lehner E, Strasser U, Lassnig E et al: A comparison between oral antiarrhythmic drugs in the prevention of atrial fibrillation after cardiac surgery: the pilot study of prevention of postoperative atrial fibrillation (SPPAF), a randomized, placebo-controlled trial. *American heart journal* 2004, 147(4):636-643.

[22] Polanczyk CA, Goldman L, Marcantonio ER, Orav EJ, Lee TH: Supraventricular arrhythmia in patients having noncardiac surgery: clinical correlates and effect on length of stay. *Annals of internal medicine* 1998, 129(4):279-285.

[23] Mariscalco G, Engstrom KG, Ferrarese S, Cozzi G, Bruno VD, Sessa F, Sala A: Relationship between atrial histopathology and atrial fibrillation after coronary bypass surgery. *The Journal of thoracic and cardiovascular surgery* 2006, 131(6):1364-1372.

[24] Schnabel RB, Sullivan LM, Levy D, Pencina MJ, Massaro JM, D'Agostino RB, Sr., Newton-Cheh C, Yamamoto JF, Magnani JW, Tadros TM et al: Development of a risk score for atrial fibrillation (Framingham Heart Study): a community-based cohort study. *Lancet* 2009, 373(9665):739-745.

[25] Passman RS, Gingold DS, Amar D, Lloyd-Jones D, Bennett CL, Zhang H, Rusch VW: Prediction rule for atrial fibrillation after major noncardiac thoracic surgery. *The Annals of thoracic surgery* 2005, 79(5):1698-1703.

[26] Verheule S, Wilson E, Everett Tt, Shanbhag S, Golden C, Olgin J: Alterations in atrial electrophysiology and tissue structure in a canine

model of chronic atrial dilatation due to mitral regurgitation. *Circulation* 2003, 107(20):2615-2622.

[27] Li D, Fareh S, Leung TK, Nattel S: Promotion of atrial fibrillation by heart failure in dogs: atrial remodeling of a different sort. *Circulation* 1999, 100(1):87-95.

[28] Barasch E, Gottdiener JS, Aurigemma G, Kitzman DW, Han J, Kop WJ, Tracy RP: Association between elevated fibrosis markers and heart failure in the elderly: the cardiovascular health study. *Circulation Heart failure* 2009, 2(4):303-310.

[29] White CM, Kluger J, Lertsburapa K, Faheem O, Coleman CI: Effect of preoperative angiotensin converting enzyme inhibitor or angiotensin receptor blocker use on the frequency of atrial fibrillation after cardiac surgery: a cohort study from the atrial fibrillation suppression trials II and III. *European journal of cardio-thoracic surgery : official journal of the European Association for Cardio-thoracic Surgery* 2007, 31(5):817-820.

[30] Shariff N, Zelenkofske S, Eid S, Weiss MJ, Mohammed MQ: Demographic determinants and effect of pre-operative angiotensin converting enzyme inhibitors and angiotensin receptor blockers on the occurrence of atrial fibrillation after CABG surgery. *BMC cardiovascular disorders* 2010, 10:7.

[31] Bruins P, te Velthuis H, Yazdanbakhsh AP, Jansen PG, van Hardevelt FW, de Beaumont EM, Wildevuur CR, Eijsman L, Trouwborst A, Hack CE: Activation of the complement system during and after cardiopulmonary bypass surgery: postsurgery activation involves C-reactive protein and is associated with postoperative arrhythmia. *Circulation* 1997, 96(10):3542-3548.

[32] Hak L, Mysliwska J, Wieckiewicz J, Szyndler K, Siebert J, Rogowski J: Interleukin-2 as a predictor of early postoperative atrial fibrillation after cardiopulmonary bypass graft (CABG). *Journal of interferon & cytokine research : the official journal of the International Society for Interferon and Cytokine Research* 2009, 29(6):327-332.

[33] Gaudino M, Andreotti F, Zamparelli R, Di Castelnuovo A, Nasso G, Burzotta F, Iacoviello L, Donati MB, Schiavello R, Maseri A *et al*: The -174G/C interleukin-6 polymorphism influences postoperative interleukin-6 levels and postoperative atrial fibrillation. Is atrial fibrillation an inflammatory complication? *Circulation* 2003, 108 Suppl 1:II195-199.

[34] Fontes ML, Mathew JP, Rinder HM, Zelterman D, Smith BR, Rinder CS: Atrial fibrillation after cardiac surgery/cardiopulmonary bypass is associated with monocyte activation. *Anesthesia and analgesia* 2005, 101(1):17-23, table of contents.

[35] Frustaci A, Chimenti C, Bellocci F, Morgante E, Russo MA, Maseri A: Histological substrate of atrial biopsies in patients with lone atrial fibrillation. *Circulation* 1997, 96(4):1180-1184.

[36] Chen MC, Chang JP, Liu WH, Yang CH, Chen YL, Tsai TH, Wang YH, Pan KL: Increased inflammatory cell infiltration in the atrial myocardium of patients with atrial fibrillation. *The American journal of cardiology* 2008, 102(7):861-865.

[37] Kumagai K, Nakashima H, Saku K: The HMG-CoA reductase inhibitor atorvastatin prevents atrial fibrillation by inhibiting inflammation in a canine sterile pericarditis model. *Cardiovascular research* 2004, 62(1):105-111.

[38] Ho KM, Tan JA: Benefits and risks of corticosteroid prophylaxis in adult cardiac surgery: a dose-response meta-analysis. *Circulation* 2009, 119(14):1853-1866.

[39] Chello M, Anselmi A, Spadaccio C, Patti G, Goffredo C, Di Sciascio G, Covino E: Simvastatin increases neutrophil apoptosis and reduces inflammatory reaction after coronary surgery. *The Annals of thoracic surgery* 2007, 83(4):1374-1380.

[40] Wagner AH, Kohler T, Ruckschloss U, Just I, Hecker M: Improvement of nitric oxide-dependent vasodilatation by HMG-CoA reductase inhibitors through attenuation of endothelial superoxide anion formation. *Arteriosclerosis, thrombosis, and vascular biology* 2000, 20(1):61-69.

[41] Workman AJ: Cardiac adrenergic control and atrial fibrillation. *Naunyn-Schmiedeberg's archives of pharmacology* 2010, 381(3):235-249.

[42] Kalman JM, Munawar M, Howes LG, Louis WJ, Buxton BF, Gutteridge G, Tonkin AM: Atrial fibrillation after coronary artery bypass grafting is associated with sympathetic activation. *The Annals of thoracic surgery* 1995, 60(6):1709-1715.

[43] Hoeldtke RD, Cilmi KM: Effects of aging on catecholamine metabolism. *The Journal of clinical endocrinology and metabolism* 1985, 60(3):479-484.

[44] Amar D, Zhang H, Miodownik S, Kadish AH: Competing autonomic mechanisms precede the onset of postoperative atrial fibrillation. *Journal of the American College of Cardiology* 2003, 42(7):1262-1268.

[45] Dimmer C, Tavernier R, Gjorgov N, Van Nooten G, Clement DL, Jordaens L: Variations of autonomic tone preceding onset of atrial fibrillation after coronary artery bypass grafting. *The American journal of cardiology* 1998, 82(1):22-25.

[46] Hogue CW, Jr., Hyder ML: Atrial fibrillation after cardiac operation: risks, mechanisms, and treatment. *The Annals of thoracic surgery* 2000, 69(1):300-306.

[47] McCord JM: Oxygen-derived free radicals in postischemic tissue injury. *The New England journal of medicine* 1985, 312(3):159-163.

[48] Kailasam R, Palin CA, Hogue CW, Jr.: Atrial fibrillation after cardiac surgery: an evidence-based approach to prevention. *Seminars in cardiothoracic and vascular anesthesia* 2005, 9(1):77-85.

[49] Carnes CA, Chung MK, Nakayama T, Nakayama H, Baliga RS, Piao S, Kanderian A, Pavia S, Hamlin RL, McCarthy PM *et al*: Ascorbate attenuates atrial pacing-induced peroxynitrite formation and electrical remodeling and decreases the incidence of postoperative atrial fibrillation. *Circulation research* 2001, 89(6):E32-38.

[50] Eslami M, Badkoubeh RS, Mousavi M, Radmehr H, Salehi M, Tavakoli N, Avadi MR: Oral ascorbic acid in combination with beta-blockers is more effective than beta-blockers alone in the prevention of atrial fibrillation after coronary artery bypass grafting. *Texas Heart Institute journal / from the Texas Heart Institute of St Luke's Episcopal Hospital, Texas Children's Hospital* 2007, 34(3):268-274.

[51] Ozaydin M, Peker O, Erdogan D, Kapan S, Turker Y, Varol E, Ozguner F, Dogan A, Ibrisim E: N-acetylcysteine for the prevention of postoperative atrial fibrillation: a prospective, randomized, placebo-controlled pilot study. *European heart journal* 2008, 29(5):625-631.

[52] Liakopoulos OJ, Choi YH, Kuhn EW, Wittwer T, Borys M, Madershahian N, Wassmer G, Wahlers T: Statins for prevention of atrial fibrillation after cardiac surgery: a systematic literature review. *The Journal of thoracic and cardiovascular surgery* 2009, 138(3):678-686 e671.

[53] Yue L, Feng J, Gaspo R, Li GR, Wang Z, Nattel S: Ionic remodeling underlying action potential changes in a canine model of atrial fibrillation. *Circulation research* 1997, 81(4):512-525.

[54] Van Wagoner DR, Pond AL, Lamorgese M, Rossie SS, McCarthy PM, Nerbonne JM: Atrial L-type Ca^{2+} currents and human atrial fibrillation. *Circulation research* 1999, 85(5):428-436.

[55] Workman AJ, Pau D, Redpath CJ, Marshall GE, Russell JA, Kane KA, Norrie J, Rankin AC: Post-operative atrial fibrillation is influenced by beta-blocker therapy but not by pre-operative atrial cellular electrophysiology. *Journal of cardiovascular electrophysiology* 2006, 17(11):1230-1238.

[56] Spach MS, Dolber PC: Relating extracellular potentials and their derivatives to anisotropic propagation at a microscopic level in human cardiac muscle. Evidence for electrical uncoupling of side-to-side fiber connections with increasing age. *Circulation research* 1986, 58(3):356-371.

[57] Goette A, Juenemann G, Peters B, Klein HU, Roessner A, Huth C, Rocken C: Determinants and consequences of atrial fibrosis in patients undergoing open heart surgery. *Cardiovascular research* 2002, 54(2):390-396.

[58] Asher CR, Miller DP, Grimm RA, Cosgrove DM, 3rd, Chung MK: Analysis of risk factors for development of atrial fibrillation early after cardiac valvular surgery. *The American journal of cardiology* 1998, 82(7):892-895.

[59] Dupont E, Ko Y, Rothery S, Coppen SR, Baghai M, Haw M, Severs NJ: The gap-junctional protein connexin40 is elevated in patients susceptible to postoperative atrial fibrillation. *Circulation* 2001, 103(6):842-849.

[60] Bradley D, Creswell LL, Hogue CW, Jr., Epstein AE, Prystowsky EN, Daoud EG: Pharmacologic prophylaxis: American College of Chest Physicians guidelines for the prevention and management of postoperative atrial fibrillation after cardiac surgery. *Chest* 2005, 128(2 Suppl):39S-47S.

[61] Ali IM, Sanalla AA, Clark V: Beta-blocker effects on postoperative atrial fibrillation. *European journal of cardio-thoracic surgery : official journal of the European Association for Cardio-thoracic Surgery* 1997, 11(6):1154-1157.

[62] Ormerod OJ, McGregor CG, Stone DL, Wisbey C, Petch MC: Arrhythmias after coronary bypass surgery. *British heart journal* 1984, 51(6):618-621.

[63] Janssen J, Loomans L, Harink J, Taams M, Brunninkhuis L, van der Starre P, Kootstra G: Prevention and treatment of supraventricular tachycardia shortly after coronary artery bypass grafting: a randomized open trial. *Angiology* 1986, 37(8):601-609.

[64] Bert AA, Reinert SE, Singh AK: A beta-blocker, not magnesium, is effective prophylaxis for atrial tachyarrhythmias after coronary artery

bypass graft surgery. *Journal of cardiothoracic and vascular anesthesia* 2001, 15(2):204-209.

[65] Mills SA, Poole GV, Jr., Breyer RH, Holliday RH, Lavender SW, 2nd, Blanton KR, Hudspeth AS, Johnston FR, Cordell AR: Digoxin and propranolol in the prophylaxis of dysrhythmias after coronary artery bypass grafting. *Circulation* 1983, 68(3 Pt 2):II222-225.

[66] Roffman J, Fieldman A: Coronary bypass-graft stenosis causing diastolic murmur in a patient on hemodialysis. *Chest* 1980, 78(2):356-357.

[67] Evrard P, Gonzalez M, Jamart J, Malhomme B, Blommaert D, Eucher P, Installe E: Prophylaxis of supraventricular and ventricular arrhythmias after coronary artery bypass grafting with low-dose sotalol. *The Annals of thoracic surgery* 2000, 70(1):151-156.

[68] Gomes JA, Ip J, Santoni-Rugiu F, Mehta D, Ergin A, Lansman S, Pe E, Newhouse TT, Chao S: Oral d,l sotalol reduces the incidence of postoperative atrial fibrillation in coronary artery bypass surgery patients: a randomized, double-blind, placebo-controlled study. *Journal of the American College of Cardiology* 1999, 34(2):334-339.

[69] Jacquet L, Evenepoel M, Marenne F, Evrard P, Verhelst R, Dion R, Goenen M: Hemodynamic effects and safety of sotalol in the prevention of supraventricular arrhythmias after coronary artery bypass surgery. *Journal of cardiothoracic and vascular anesthesia* 1994, 8(4):431-436.

[70] Matsuura K, Takahara Y, Sudo Y, Ishida K: Effect of Sotalol in the prevention of atrial fibrillation following coronary artery bypass grafting. *The Japanese journal of thoracic and cardiovascular surgery : official publication of the Japanese Association for Thoracic Surgery = Nihon Kyobu Geka Gakkai zasshi* 2001, 49(10):614-617.

[71] Pfisterer ME, Kloter-Weber UC, Huber M, Osswald S, Buser PT, Skarvan K, Stulz PM: Prevention of supraventricular tachyarrhythmias after open heart operation by low-dose sotalol: a prospective, double-blind, randomized, placebo-controlled study. *The Annals of thoracic surgery* 1997, 64(4):1113-1119.

[72] Weber UK, Osswald S, Buser P, Huber M, Skarvan K, Stulz P, Pfisterer M: Significance of Supraventricular Tachyarrhythmias After Coronary Artery Bypass Graft Surgery and Their Prevention by Low-Dose Sotalol: A Prospective Double-Blind Randomized Placebo-Controlled Study. *Journal of cardiovascular pharmacology and therapeutics* 1998, 3(3):209-216.

[73] Parikka H, Toivonen L, Heikkila L, Virtanen K, Jarvinen A: Comparison of sotalol and metoprolol in the prevention of atrial fibrillation after coronary artery bypass surgery. *Journal of cardiovascular pharmacology* 1998, 31(1):67-73.

[74] Suttorp MJ, Kingma JH, Tjon Joe Gin RM, van Hemel NM, Koomen EM, Defauw JA, Adan AJ, Ernst SM: Efficacy and safety of low- and high-dose sotalol versus propranolol in the prevention of supraventricular tachyarrhythmias early after coronary artery bypass operations. *The Journal of thoracic and cardiovascular surgery* 1990, 100(6):921-926.

[75] Butler J, Harriss DR, Sinclair M, Westaby S: Amiodarone prophylaxis for tachycardias after coronary artery surgery: a randomised, double blind, placebo controlled trial. *British heart journal* 1993, 70(1):56-60.

[76] Daoud EG, Strickberger SA, Man KC, Goyal R, Deeb GM, Bolling SF, Pagani FD, Bitar C, Meissner MD, Morady F: Preoperative amiodarone as prophylaxis against atrial fibrillation after heart surgery. *The New England journal of medicine* 1997, 337(25):1785-1791.

[77] Dorge H, Schoendube FA, Schoberer M, Stellbrink C, Voss M, Messmer BJ: Intraoperative amiodarone as prophylaxis against atrial fibrillation after coronary operations. *The Annals of thoracic surgery* 2000, 69(5):1358-1362.

[78] Giri S, White CM, Dunn AB, Felton K, Freeman-Bosco L, Reddy P, Tsikouris JP, Wilcox HA, Kluger J: Oral amiodarone for prevention of atrial fibrillation after open heart surgery, the Atrial Fibrillation Suppression Trial (AFIST): a randomised placebo-controlled trial. *Lancet* 2001, 357(9259):830-836.

[79] Guarnieri T, Nolan S, Gottlieb SO, Dudek A, Lowry DR: Intravenous amiodarone for the prevention of atrial fibrillation after open heart surgery: the Amiodarone Reduction in Coronary Heart (ARCH) trial. *Journal of the American College of Cardiology* 1999, 34(2):343-347.

[80] Hohnloser SH, Meinertz T, Dammbacher T, Steiert K, Jahnchen E, Zehender M, Fraedrich G, Just H: Electrocardiographic and antiarrhythmic effects of intravenous amiodarone: results of a prospective, placebo-controlled study. *American heart journal* 1991, 121(1 Pt 1):89-95.

[81] Lee SH, Chang CM, Lu MJ, Lee RJ, Cheng JJ, Hung CR, Chen SA: Intravenous amiodarone for prevention of atrial fibrillation after coronary artery bypass grafting. *The Annals of thoracic surgery* 2000, 70(1):157-161.

[82] Maras D, Boskovic SD, Popovic Z, Neskovic AN, Kovacevic S, Otasevic P, Marinkovic J, Vuk L, Borzanovic M, Nastasic S et al: Single-day loading dose of oral amiodarone for the prevention of new-onset atrial fibrillation after coronary artery bypass surgery. *American heart journal* 2001, 141(5):E8.

[83] Treggiari-Venzi MM, Waeber JL, Perneger TV, Suter PM, Adamec R, Romand JA: Intravenous amiodarone or magnesium sulphate is not cost-beneficial prophylaxis for atrial fibrillation after coronary artery bypass surgery. *British journal of anaesthesia* 2000, 85(5):690-695.

[84] Solomon AJ, Greenberg MD, Kilborn MJ, Katz NM: Amiodarone versus a beta-blocker to prevent atrial fibrillation after cardiovascular surgery. *American heart journal* 2001, 142(5):811-815.

[85] Ferraris VA, Ferraris SP, Gilliam H, Berry W: Verapamil prophylaxis for postoperative atrial dysrhythmias: a prospective, randomized, double-blind study using drug level monitoring. *The Annals of thoracic surgery* 1987, 43(5):530-533.

[86] Davison R, Hartz R, Kaplan K, Parker M, Feiereisel P, Michaelis L: Prophylaxis of supraventricular tachyarrhythmia after coronary bypass surgery with oral verapamil: a randomized, double-blind trial. *The Annals of thoracic surgery* 1985, 39(4):336-339.

[87] Smith EE, Shore DF, Monro JL, Ross JK: Oral verapamil fails to prevent supraventricular tachycardia following coronary artery surgery. *International journal of cardiology* 1985, 9(1):37-44.

[88] Williams DB, Misbach GA, Kruse AP, Ivey TD: Oral verapamil for prophylaxis of supraventricular tachycardia after myocardial revascularization. A randomized trial. *The Journal of thoracic and cardiovascular surgery* 1985, 90(4):592-596.

[89] Chee TP, Prakash NS, Desser KB, Benchimol A: Postoperative supraventricular arrhythmias and the role of prophylactic digoxin in cardiac surgery. *American heart journal* 1982, 104(5 Pt 1):974-977.

[90] Csicsko JF, Schatzlein MH, King RD: Immediate postoperative digitalization in the prophylaxis of supraventricular arrhythmias following coronary artery bypass. *The Journal of thoracic and cardiovascular surgery* 1981, 81(3):419-422.

[91] Johnson LW, Dickstein RA, Fruehan CT, Kane P, Potts JL, Smulyan H, Webb WR, Eich RH: Prophylactic digitalization for coronary artery bypass surgery. *Circulation* 1976, 53(5):819-822.

[92] Parker FB, Jr., Greiner-Hayes C, Bove EL, Marvasti MA, Johnson LW, Eich RH: Supraventricular arrhythmias following coronary artery

bypass. The effect of preoperative digitalis. *The Journal of thoracic and cardiovascular surgery* 1983, 86(4):594-600.

[93] Weiner B, Rheinlander HF, Decker EL, Cleveland RJ: Digoxin prophylaxis following coronary artery bypass surgery. *Clinical pharmacy* 1986, 5(1):55-58.

[94] Tyras DH, Stothert JC, Jr., Kaiser GC, Barner HB, Codd JE, Willman VL: Supraventricular tachyarrhythmias after myocardial revascularization: a randomized trial of prophylactic digitalization. *The Journal of thoracic and cardiovascular surgery* 1979, 77(2):310-314.

[95] Toraman F, Karabulut EH, Alhan HC, Dagdelen S, Tarcan S: Magnesium infusion dramatically decreases the incidence of atrial fibrillation after coronary artery bypass grafting. *The Annals of thoracic surgery* 2001, 72(4):1256-1261; discussion 1261-1252.

[96] Yeatman M, Caputo M, Narayan P, Lotto AA, Ascione R, Bryan AJ, Angelini GD: Magnesium-supplemented warm blood cardioplegia in patients undergoing coronary artery revascularization. *The Annals of thoracic surgery* 2002, 73(1):112-118.

[97] Goldman L: Supraventricular tachyarrhythmias in hospitalized adults after surgery. Clinical correlates in patients over 40 years of age after major noncardiac surgery. *Chest* 1978, 73(4):450-454.

[98] Walsh SR, Oates JE, Anderson JA, Blair SD, Makin CA, Walsh CJ: Postoperative arrhythmias in colorectal surgical patients: incidence and clinical correlates. *Colorectal disease : the official journal of the Association of Coloproctology of Great Britain and Ireland* 2006, 8(3):212-216.

[99] Vaporciyan AA, Correa AM, Rice DC, Roth JA, Smythe WR, Swisher SG, Walsh GL, Putnam JB, Jr.: Risk factors associated with atrial fibrillation after noncardiac thoracic surgery: analysis of 2588 patients. *The Journal of thoracic and cardiovascular surgery* 2004, 127(3):779-786.

[100] Harpole DH, Liptay MJ, DeCamp MM, Jr., Mentzer SJ, Swanson SJ, Sugarbaker DJ: Prospective analysis of pneumonectomy: risk factors for major morbidity and cardiac dysrhythmias. *The Annals of thoracic surgery* 1996, 61(3):977-982.

[101] Park BJ, Zhang H, Rusch VW, Amar D: Video-assisted thoracic surgery does not reduce the incidence of postoperative atrial fibrillation after pulmonary lobectomy. *The Journal of thoracic and cardiovascular surgery* 2007, 133(3):775-779.

[102] Krowka MJ, Pairolero PC, Trastek VF, Payne WS, Bernatz PE: Cardiac dysrhythmia following pneumonectomy. Clinical correlates and prognostic significance. *Chest* 1987, 91(4):490-495.

[103] Curtis JJ, Parker BM, McKenney CA, Wagner-Mann CC, Walls JT, Demmy TL, Schmaltz RA: Incidence and predictors of supraventricular dysrhythmias after pulmonary resection. *The Annals of thoracic surgery* 1998, 66(5):1766-1771.

[104] Konno O, Tezuka T, Muto A, Hoshino Y, Kogure M, Koyama S, Suzuki H, Inoue H, Motoki R: [Postoperative arrhythmia after operation of esophageal cancer]. *[Zasshi] [Journal] Nihon Kyobu Geka Gakkai* 1993, 41(1):45-51.

[105] Stippel DL, Taylan C, Schroder W, Beckurts KT, Holscher AH: Supraventricular tachyarrhythmia as early indicator of a complicated course after esophagectomy. *Diseases of the esophagus : official journal of the International Society for Diseases of the Esophagus / ISDE* 2005, 18(4):267-273.

[106] Tisdale JE, Wroblewski HA, Kesler KA: Prophylaxis of atrial fibrillation after noncardiac thoracic surgery. *Seminars in thoracic and cardiovascular surgery* 2010, 22(4):310-320.

[107] Sohn GH, Shin DH, Byun KM, Han HJ, Cho SJ, Song YB, Kim JH, On YK, Kim JS: The incidence and predictors of postoperative atrial fibrillation after noncardiothoracic surgery. *Korean Circ J* 2009, 39(3):100-104.

[108] Christians KK, Wu B, Quebbeman EJ, Brasel KJ: Postoperative atrial fibrillation in noncardiothoracic surgical patients. *American journal of surgery* 2001, 182(6):713-715.

[109] Onaitis M, D'Amico T, Zhao Y, O'Brien S, Harpole D: Risk factors for atrial fibrillation after lung cancer surgery: analysis of the Society of Thoracic Surgeons general thoracic surgery database. *The Annals of thoracic surgery* 2010, 90(2):368-374.

[110] Roselli EE, Murthy SC, Rice TW, Houghtaling PL, Pierce CD, Karchmer DP, Blackstone EH: Atrial fibrillation complicating lung cancer resection. *The Journal of thoracic and cardiovascular surgery* 2005, 130(2):438-444.

[111] Nojiri T, Maeda H, Takeuchi Y, Funakoshi Y, Kimura T, Maekura R, Yamamoto K, Okumura M: Predictive value of B-type natriuretic peptide for postoperative atrial fibrillation following pulmonary resection for lung cancer. *European journal of cardio-thoracic surgery :*

official journal of the European Association for Cardio-thoracic Surgery 2010, 37(4):787-791.

[112] Amar D, Roistacher N, Burt M, Reinsel RA, Ginsberg RJ, Wilson RS: Clinical and echocardiographic correlates of symptomatic tachydysrhythmias after noncardiac thoracic surgery. *Chest* 1995, 108(2):349-354.

[113] Amar D, Zhang H, Heerdt PM, Park B, Fleisher M, Thaler HT: Statin use is associated with a reduction in atrial fibrillation after noncardiac thoracic surgery independent of C-reactive protein. *Chest* 2005, 128(5):3421-3427.

[114] Jakobsen CJ, Bille S, Ahlburg P, Rybro L, Hjortholm K, Andresen EB: Perioperative metoprolol reduces the frequency of atrial fibrillation after thoracotomy for lung resection. *Journal of cardiothoracic and vascular anesthesia* 1997, 11(6):746-751.

[115] Bayliff CD, Massel DR, Inculet RI, Malthaner RA, Quinton SD, Powell FS, Kennedy RS: Propranolol for the prevention of postoperative arrhythmias in general thoracic surgery. *The Annals of thoracic surgery* 1999, 67(1):182-186.

[116] Amar D, Roistacher N, Burt ME, Rusch VW, Bains MS, Leung DH, Downey RJ, Ginsberg RJ: Effects of diltiazem versus digoxin on dysrhythmias and cardiac function after pneumonectomy. *The Annals of thoracic surgery* 1997, 63(5):1374-1381; discussion 1381-1372.

[117] Amar D, Roistacher N, Rusch VW, Leung DH, Ginsburg I, Zhang H, Bains MS, Downey RJ, Korst RJ, Ginsberg RJ: Effects of diltiazem prophylaxis on the incidence and clinical outcome of atrial arrhythmias after thoracic surgery. *The Journal of thoracic and cardiovascular surgery* 2000, 120(4):790-798.

[118] Van Mieghem W, Tits G, Demuynck K, Lacquet L, Deneffe G, Tjandra-Maga T, Demedts M: Verapamil as prophylactic treatment for atrial fibrillation after lung operations. *The Annals of thoracic surgery* 1996, 61(4):1083-1085; discussion 1086.

[119] Lindgren L, Lepantalo M, von Knorring J, Rosenberg P, Orko R, Scheinin B: Effect of verapamil on right ventricular pressure and atrial tachyarrhythmia after thoracotomy. *British journal of anaesthesia* 1991, 66(2):205-211.

[120] Lanza LA, Visbal AI, DeValeria PA, Zinsmeister AR, Diehl NN, Trastek VF: Low-dose oral amiodarone prophylaxis reduces atrial fibrillation after pulmonary resection. *The Annals of thoracic surgery* 2003, 75(1):223-230; discussion 230.

[121] Terzi A, Furlan G, Chiavacci P, Dal Corso B, Luzzani A, Dalla Volta S: Prevention of atrial tachyarrhythmias after non-cardiac thoracic surgery by infusion of magnesium sulfate. *The Thoracic and cardiovascular surgeon* 1996, 44(6):300-303.

In: General and Abdominal Surgery
Editor: Kassandra Sarah Slavomir

ISBN: 978-1-63117-440-7
© 2014 Nova Science Publishers, Inc.

Chapter 4

Perioperative Period, Stress Response, Immune Suppression and Cancer Recurrence

***M. F. Ramirez, P. Tran and Juan P. Cata**[*]*
Department of Anesthesiology and Perioperative Medicine,
University of Texas-MD Anderson Cancer Center,
Houston, Texas - US

Abstract

During the perioperative of any major surgery, there is an intense activation of the sympathetic nervous system, the hypothalamus-pituitary-adrenal axis, and several cellular and soluble components of the inflammatory cascade. All together elements are part so-called stress response. Two characteristics of an exaggerated and uncontrolled stress response are exhaustion and immune suppression. This last, in particular, is relevant in the context of cancer surgery because can lead to growth of any potential postoperative minimal residual disease. To complicate more this matter, anesthetics, opioids and blood transfusions can also contribute to the so-called perioperative immune suppression and cancer

[*] Corresponding author: Juan P. Cata, MD, Department of Anesthesiology and Perioperative Medicine, Unit 0408, The University of Texas MD Anderson Cancer Center, 1515 Holcombe Boulevard, Houston, TX 77030 USA, Email: jcata@mdanderson.org, Telephone: 713-792-4582, Fax: 713-745-2956

growth. Hence, surgeons and anesthesiologist have tried to developed pharmacological and non-pharmacological interventions targeted to avoid the unwanted effects of an exaggerated stress response.

Introduction

Surgery is still the main treatment option for a variety of cancers. Depending on the magnitude and duration of the surgical insult, the body undergoes a series of metabolic, neuroendocrine, immune and inflammatory changes leading to healing and restoration of homeostasis. An increase in the circulating concentrations of catecholamines, cortisol, angiogenic factors and inflammatory mediators such as prostaglandin E is the signature of the stress response but unfortunately an exaggerated release of those mediators may tilt the balance towards uncontrolled inflammation and immune suppression. In the context of cancer, this immunosuppression may lead to accelerated tumor growth and metastasis formation. Hence, it has been indicated that one of the main roles of the physicians during the perioperative period is to minimize the stress response and immune suppression associated to surgery. Minimally invasive surgery, regional anesthesia and pharmacological interventions including the use of corticosteroids, beta-blockers and non-steroidal anti-inflammatory drugs have been tried in different surgical settings with the goal of ameliorate stress, the inflammatory response and immune suppression associated to surgery. Unfortunately, the results of the studies evaluating those interventions are mixed. The purpose of this chapter is to provide evidence between stress response and perioperative strategies targeted to minimize immune suppression with the goal of reducing tumor growth and metastasis formation.

Surgical Stress

Stress can be defined as any insult that will cause harm to the body and disrupt its ability to function or reach homeostasis. Each patient will respond to the stress in different ways based on the characteristics of the insult and her/his co-morbidities (heart failure, diabetes, liver failure), and genetic predispositions. All of these factors not only influence the surgical stress response but might lead to a maladaptive stress response [1, 2]. The host response to surgery is an amplification of the responses that are activated under stress. The initial insult leads to local and generalized inflammation with the activation of the neuroendocrine system characterized by a marked increase in catecholamines and other stress hormones to produce a hyper metabolic-catabolic state [1]. The hormonal induced metabolic response produces a marked increase in energy demands that the body must respond by mobilizing energy and nutrient and activating the body's defenses to protect itself from stressor.

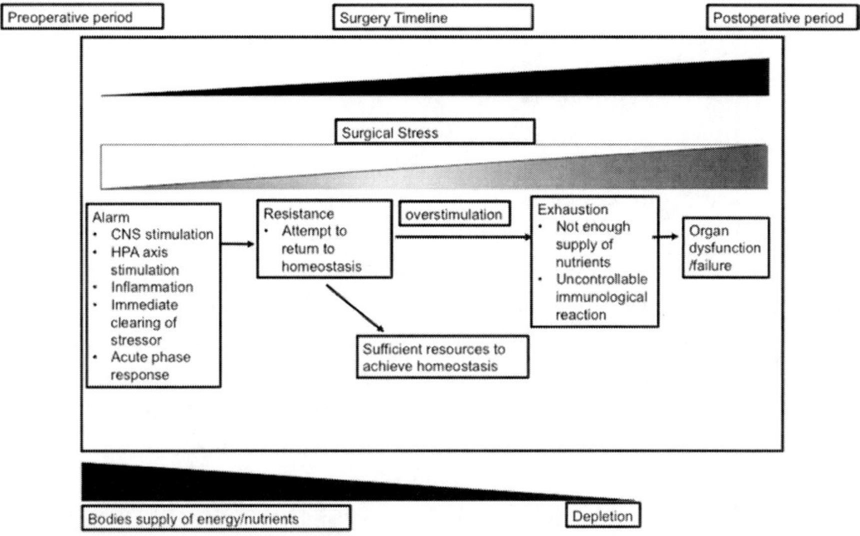

Figure 1. Perioperative stress-response.

The concept of the stress response of the general adaptation is broken down into multiple phases: the alarm phase, the resistance phase, and exhaustion phase, which are depicted in Figure 1 [3, 4]. After surgical trauma the first response is *alarm phase*, the basic purpose of this stage is to prepare the body for immediate action: energy is mobilized to cope with emergency. Epinephrine is the dominant hormone of the alarm phase. The *resistance phase* follows the alarm phase as an attempt of the body to return to homeostasis. This phase is where the overall metabolism in the body is dedicated to provide maximum amount of energy and nutrients for the response. Glucocorticoids are the dominant hormone of the resistance phase. If the stressor is removed and the body is able maintain it-self, it will go into the *recovery phase*. As time progresses the body will continue to utilize its resources and will utilize its reserves until it is expended. An exaggerated stress response will increase the use of energy expenditure that might continue until it reaches the stage of *exhaustion*. This is characterized by the insufficient supply of nutrients to continue the stress response with an uncontrollable immunological and inflammatory reaction [3, 4].

The body has multiple mechanisms to recover and respond in order to achieve homeostasis. The main pathways the body applies are the acute phase response, the hypothalamic-pituitary axis response, and the sympathetic response.

Sympathetic Response

As any incision is made to the patient, there are nociceptors that are activated leading to activation of the peripheral sensory nerves. All of the afferent nerves transmit the signal through the spinal cord to the thalamus. As the site of trauma is still exposed, there is a constant stimulation of pain being perceived [5]. The thalamus plays a role in relaying sensory and motor cortex signals to the hypothalamus. Then, the sympathetic response is created by the adrenal medulla and sympathetic nerves that release catecholamines such as epinephrine and norepinephrine, respectively [6].

In general terms, catecholamines increase the metabolic rate, in a predominant catabolic state and stimulate the nervous system to increase alertness. The effects of epinephrine and norepinephrine are short lasting but the continual release of the catecholamines allows a constant response [7-9]. Blood glucose concentrations are related to the intensity of surgery due to the increased amount of catecholamines during surgical stress and remain high [10]. Catecholamines facilitate glucose production as a result of hepatic glycogenlysis and gluconeogenesis. Protein breakdown is increased and as a result skeletal muscle and some visceral protein is catabolized in order to provide energy as well as amino acids to synthesize other proteins associated with the stress response [11].

Endocrine Response

Hypothalamic-Pituitary-Adrenal Axis

The activation of the hypothalamus leads to the action of the hypothalamic-pituitary-adrenal axis. The overall endocrine response is to increase metabolism to provide energy sources for repair and survival. The hypothalamus activates the release of hormones of the anterior pituitary in an indirect fashion by the use of hormone releasing factors [12].

Adrenocorticotropic hormone (ACTH) from the anterior pituitary stimulates the adrenal cortex to release cortisol. Similar to the catecholamines, cortisol is a metabolic hormone that favors production of energy sources in the breakdown of fats, proteins, and the synthesis of glucose by glycogenesis and gluconeogenesis. ACTH and cortisol has been show to increases very rapidly at the start of surgery [9]. Usually a feedback mechanism operates so that increase levels of cortisol inhibit further the secretion of ACTH, however this control mechanism is ineffective after and during surgery so both of these hormones remain high leading to hyperglycemia and overstimulation of the organs leading to exhaustion of nutrients [13, 14].

Cortisol also has a major role in the anti-inflammatory activity [15]. It inhibits the accumulation of macrophages and neutrophils to the areas of inflammation and interferes with the synthesis of inflammatory mediators such as prostaglandins leading to immunosuppressive effects [14].

The Acute Phase Response

The local response to tissue injury is inflammation which is characterized by vasodilation in order to allow pro-inflammatory mediators such as leukocytes to rush upon the site [11, 16]. The goals of this phase are: 1) to contain any infectious agents by the generation of superoxides by phagocytes mainly to kill invading microorganisms; however, the production of exaggerated quantities of superoxides might lead, in fact, to further damage [17, 18] and 2) to begin repairing of tissue damage.

Activated leukocytes, fibroblasts, and damaged/exposed endothelial cells immediately being to synthesize and release cytokines which play a major role in maintaining the inflammatory response. The major cytokines that are released to mediate the inflammatory response are interleukin 1 (IL-1), tumor necrosis factor a (TNF-α), and interleukin 8 [19]. There are released and act as a positive feedback mechanism to elicit a stronger response. These cytokines may also play a role to mediate fever [20]. The amount of cytokine released is reflected on the magnitude of the trauma. Cytokines released from the site of injury then travel to the liver in order to activate the acute phase response. The acute phase response results in the production of acute phase proteins, complement factors, neuroendocrine mediators which aid in tissue repair [1]. The acute phase proteins include C-reactive protein, fibrinogen, haptoglobin, immunosuppressive acidic protein, and anti-proteinases. As the production of acute phase proteins increase, concentrations of other proteins produced in in the liver decrease such as albumin [21]. It also leads to increase of granulocytes and platelets which activate the complement and coagulation pathways but a decrease in levels of lymphocytes [9, 22]. Similar to the sympathetic and the hypothalamic-pituitary-adrenal response, the acute phase response also induces a catabolic state and favors the production of more glucose and free amino acids. The cytokines interleukin 6 (IL-6), interleukin 1 (IL-1) and TNF-α, and the prostaglandins that are in circulation can induce fever by acting upon the hypothalamus which is activated by prostanglandins, causing a higher thermoregulatory set point [23-25].

Prostaglandins are immediately released upon activation of the inflammatory response and are released before recruitment of leukocytes and infiltration of immune cells augmenting arterial dilation, increasing vascular permeability, and inducing hyperalgesia [26]. In addition of increasing the immune/inflammatory response, other types of prostaglandins are produced to function as an anti-inflammatory to prevent overstimulation of the prostaglandins in the inflammatory response [16].

The Immune System

The immune system protects the host from tumor development by activating and modulating a complex system of cell and soluble mediators. Among the soluble mediators, we can include prostaglandins, growth factors, and interleukins. Interferon-γ, IL-1α, and IL-2 can induce cancer cell death directly but most importantly, the latter mediator can amplify cell-mediated immunity which includes natural killer cells (NK cells), cytotoxic lymphocytes (CD8), NK-T cell lymphocytes, antigens presenting cells (APC), and helper lymphocytes (Th) [27, 28]. The action of CD4 T helper is classified according to the role and pattern of the cytokines they secrete. For instance, the Th1 cell response is characterized by the production of interferon-alpha (IFN-α), IL-2, and tumor necrosis factor (TNF-α) and it is highly effective in enhancing cellular immunity necessary for tumor cell destruction. In contrast, the Th2 cell response produces IL-4, IL-5, IL-10, and IL-13, which mediate humoral response and promote tumor growth [27]. To complicate this matter, the Th1/Th2 balance is predominant towards Th2 after cancer surgery as a result of a decrease in Th1 and increase in Th2 response [29, 30].

In general, catecholamines, glucocorticoids and inflammation leads to depression of the cell mediated response against cancer [9, 31-33]. Prolonged and exaggerated stress will cause an overstimulation of the Th2 cytokines to counterbalance the continual inflammation which will eventually contribute to even more to depression in the immune system [34, 35].

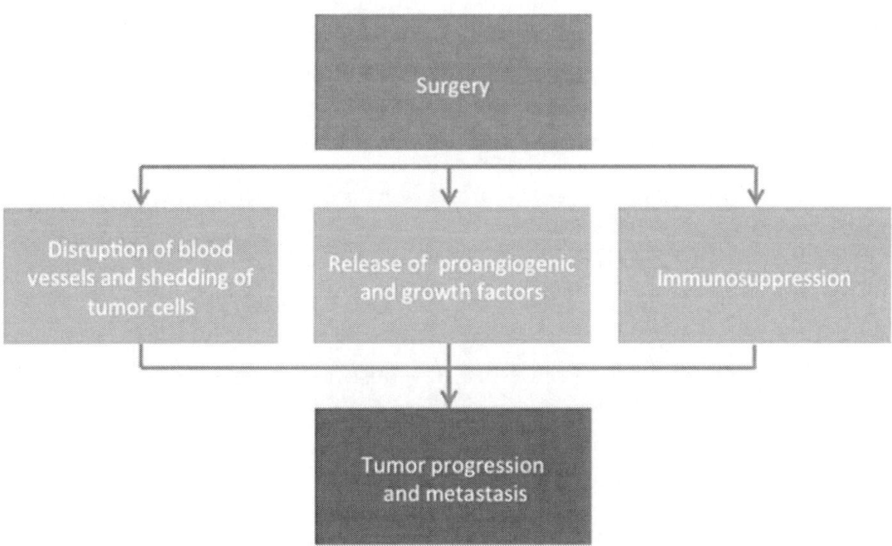

Figure 2. Potential mechanisms of surgery-induced tumor progression.

The surgical approach to cancer patients should have a special consideration by the surgeon because this patient population characteristically presents some unique characteristics that must be taken into account to approach, intervene, and, perhaps, decrease the short (infection and sepsis) and long-term (cancer recurrence and metastasis) consequences of surgery. The goals of cancer surgery include complete tumor resection, preservation of the anatomy and functionality of the affected organ, improvement of quality of life, diagnosis, and staging. Unfortunately, there is growing evidence that has shown that cancer surgery *per se* is a risk factor for the spreading, establishment, and recurrence of malignancy [36]. Several possible mechanisms have been suggested as the protumoral effect of surgery (Figure 2). First, during cancer surgery the removal of tumor is characterized by disruption of the integrity of blood vessels feeding the tumor, and this disarrangement promotes the shedding of the tumor cells through the systemic circulation [37-39]. Secondly, tumor manipulation stimulates the release of pro angiogenic and growth factors which favors growth and metastasis [40]. Fourth, surgical stress, together with subsequent metabolic, neuroendocrine, and inflammatory response results in a significant impairment of the cell-mediated immunity against cancer [41-44]. Cancer patients might suffer from significant immunosuppression that is explained by the cancer itself, chemotherapy, radiotherapy, and malnutrition. Additionally, an aspect inherent to surgery, such as general anesthesia and analgesic drugs, may also play a role in metastasis, because they are also immune suppressive[45, 46]. All these mechanisms occurring at the same time may have a synergic effect in promoting cancer surgery prognosis.

Response to Surgical Stress and Tumor Progression

The relationship between stress response and progression of neoplastic disease has been described for several types of cancers. The mechanisms by which the stress response contributes to tumor progression include activation of the sympathetic nervous system, activation of the hypothalamic-pituitary adrenal axis, and promotion of inflammation [41-44, 47].

nportant to confirm whether such interventions lead to improve long-term
ival although initial data in animals and in human appear to be promising.

cocorticoids

Glucocorticoids (GC) are traditionally known for their suppressive action
the immune system [61]. Specifically, surgery increases corticosterone
ls and this increase is negatively correlated with NK cell function [62].
eover, glucocorticoids down-regulates the secretion of cytokines IL-1β,
, *IL-4, IL-6, IL-8, IL-12, IFN–γ and up-regulates the secretion IL-10 and*
⁷–α [63]. Hence, their overall effect appears to be a disruption of the
/Th2 balance towards a predominant Th2 response [29, 30].
cocorticoids have been widely used in cancer therapy for the treatment of
symptoms caused by the tumor including inflammation, edema and pain
·67]. Dexamethasone is extensively used in different types of surgery.
mal studies have suggested that the administration of GC during the
operative period can exert anti tumoral effects [68]. The administration of
amethasone on animals with pancreatic cancer can inhibit the expression of
·inflammatory cytokines and invasiveness of malignant cells in vitro,
itionally dexamethasone decreases the size of the recurrent tumor and also
inished the number of metastases after surgical resection [68]. By the other
d, other authors have shown in *in vitro* models that dexamethasone
resses the function of the NK cells and that the perioperative
iinistration may therefore augment tumor recurrence after cancer surgery
70]. Based on this preclinical data, human studies have been conducted to
:idate the association between systemic dexamethasone administration (4 to
mg) and tumor recurrence in cancer patient who underwent surgery for
rian cancer. Unfortunately, De Oliveira et al. did not find evidence for an
)ciation between perioperative systemic dexamethasone administration and
rian cancer recurrence [71]. Therefore, it is unclear whether or not the
operative administration of dexamethasone is associated with cancer
irrence and metastasis.

)stanglandins

A relationship between chronic inflammation and cancer has been
posed by many authors [72-74]. The enzymes responsible for the

Catecholamines

So far, two models have been proposed to explain the pr
of adrenergic stimulation during surgery. The first mod
activation of beta-adrenergic receptors that promotes angiogei
and proliferation of cancer cells [48-50]. For example, e
norepinephrine appears to increase the *in vitro* invasive poter
growth of ovarian cancer cells [51]. Additionally, the stimula
adrenergic receptor in prostatic and breast cancer protects ca
apoptosis [52, 53]. The second model proposes that adrene
suppresses the cell-mediated response against cancer c
Specifically, beta adrenergic stimulation suppresses the activi
macrophages, and dendritic cells [56], shifts the Th1/Th2 balai
cell-mediated response with Th2 predominance [57].

It is now recognized that attenuation of the surgical stres
beta-blockers could be a possible strategy to decrease the risl
Benish et al. suggested that the use of beta-blocker with COX
rats during the perioperative period improved immune c
reduced the risk of tumor metastasis [58]. Furthermore, the au
the administration of the drug during 3 days before surgery y
beneficial effect as a single pre- operative dose administrat
available clinical evidence suggests a protective effect of chror
and cancer survival, today there is no RCT completed availabl
of this agent during the perioperative period and long-to
Although, few studies have shown that patients taking beta
higher survival and lower recurrence and metastasis, all their e
based on retrospective data analysis which suffers from signi
biases. Specifically the chronic use of beta-blockers in triple
cancer patients before surgery is associated with improved
survival [59]. In the case of patient with diagnosis of non- s
cancer with metastasis, the use of beta-blocker during chei
associated with an improved overall survival [60].

To date, there is no evidence demonstrating that the use o
perioperative regimen of COX 2 inhibitor and beta-blockers in
modified survival. Only one RCT (NCT00502684) is now be
with the purpose to examine if the perioperative adminis
combination of beta-blockers together with COX 2 inhibitor
suppression of cellular immunity and decrease cancer recurren

production of PGs are referred to as cyclooxygenase (COX). PGE2, in particular, may contribute to the cancer process through one or more mechanisms including cell proliferation, apoptosis, adhesion, invasion, and angiogenesis [75]. Additionally, there is data that have shown PGE2 to inhibit the cytotoxicity of NK cells, reduce the CD4 lymphocyte survival, and prevent the activation of CD8 lymphocytes [76-78]. Human results from experimental studies have shown that COX-2 is highly expressed in solid malignancies including breast, colon, prostate, lung, pancreas, and skin cancer [79-81]. The potential role of COX enzymes in preinvasive stages of breast cancer tumorigenesis has been investigated because of previous human epidemiological studies indicating an association between the use of non-steroidal anti-inflammatory drugs (NSAIDs) and a decreased risk of breast cancer. Overexpression of COX-2 been correlated with progression of ductal carcinoma in situ to invasive breast carcinoma [82]. It has also been suggested that the elevated PGs production can be used as marker of high metastatic potential for neoplastic cells in breast cancer [83]. The role of PGs and COX enzyme has also been evaluated in colon cancer. Human colon cancer tissue produces more PGE2 than surrounding normal tissue. Moreover, PGE2 production results in activation of a signaling pathway that promotes cell proliferation and inhibits cell death. COX-2 is progressively overexpressed during the step sequence from adenoma to carcinoma [84].

During the last decades, there has been a particular interest in the use of NSAIDs not only for the symptomatic treatment but also for additional therapeutic component of the standard of care for cancer patients. Most of the work, experimental and clinical, relating COX-2 to cancer involve colon cancer, breast cancer and, to a lesser extent, gastric and esophageal cancer [85]. In regards to experimental evidence, COX-2 selective inhibitors like celecoxib has shown to block tumor growth and number and size of metastasis in animal models of lung cancer and colon cancer by decreasing angiogenesis [86]. Likewise, Harris et al. evaluated the anti-tumor effect of celecoxib in an animal model with breast cancer [87]. Investigation conducted by Everson et al., suggested that regular aspirin intake produced an important reduction in lung, colon and breast cancer risk [88]. Subsequently some other authors have shown the protective effect of COX-2 inhibition in the development of lung cancer [89, 90]. Additionally, a meta-analysis found that regular intake of NSAIDs (primarily aspirin and ibuprofen) was associated with a reduced risk of developing colon (63%), lung (36%), breast (36%), and prostate (39%) cancer [91]. Very little clinical data exist regarding the use of COX-2 inhibition during the perioperative period and cancer recurrence. A study on the postoperative survival of patients given a daily dose of aspirin (25-50 mg/day) after resection for squamous cell carcinoma of the esophagus or adenocarcinoma of the cardia showed an improvement in 5-year survival rate for all patients on aspirin with T2N0M0 esophageal cancer [92]. Pre-surgical treatment with COX-2 inhibitors, on the other hand, appears to be another interesting strategy to approach surgical patients. Unfortunately, the data regarding the use of preoperative COX-2 inhibitors only refers to the histological changes in breast and prostatic cancer and not to the magnitude of this intervention on cancer recurrence and survival[93, 94].

Anesthesia/Analgesia and Tumor Progression

It has been well-documented in *in vitro* and *in vivo* animal models that anesthetics and analgesics could modify the immune response during surgery (Figure 3). For instance, the intravenous anesthetic/analgesic ketamine and thiopental decrease the function of NK cells and promote the release of pro-inflammatory cytokines which ultimately promotes immunosuppression and distant metastasis [45, 95, 96]. On the contrary, propofol lacks the negative effect on the immune function of intravenous anesthetics and, in fact, this agent has been suggested to decrease the metastatic potential of tumor cells since propofol preserves the function of NK cells and Th1/Th2 balance [45]. Not only intravenous anesthetics have been implicated in this theory; volatile anesthetics have shown to have a similar behavior in regards to immunosuppression [46, 97]. Additionally, opioids have been suggested to contribute to tumor progression by enhancing proliferation of endothelial cells in breast cancer and glioblastoma multiforme models[98, 99]. Furthermore, opioids appear to favor the Th2 response [100, 101].

The potential ability of regional anesthesia to improve the long-term prognosis after cancer surgery could be explained by two different mechanisms. First, regional anesthesia attenuates surgery stress response [102]. Second, patients who undergo surgery under regional anesthesia requires less opioids, intravenous anesthetics and volatiles anesthetics which could result in less immunosuppression and more efficient defense against tumor progression[36]. The effect of regional anesthesia on oncological outcomes in human studies is conflicting.

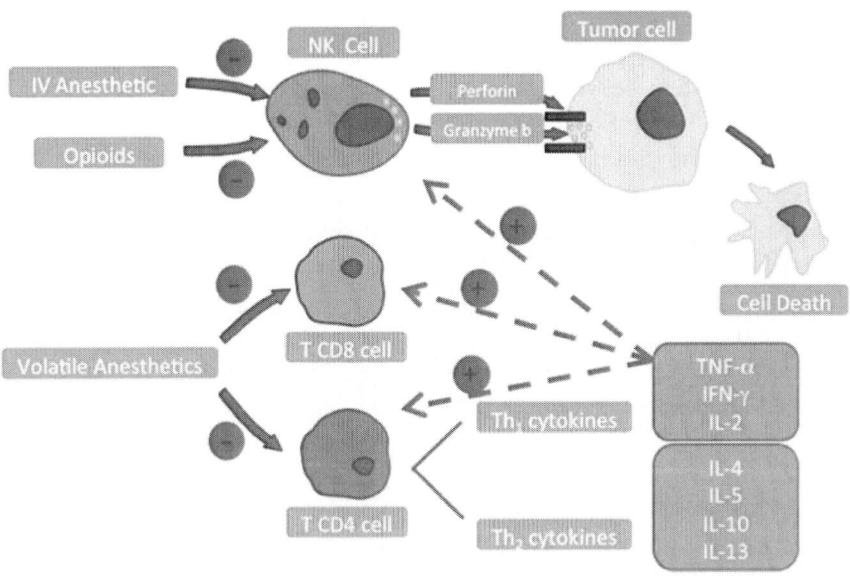

Figure 3. Potential mechanisms of anesthetics/analgesics induced immune suppression.

The first clinical evidence was a study in which breast cancer patients underwent surgery under sevoflurane-opioids or propofol-paravertebral blockade. Paravertebral anesthesia and analgesia for breast cancer surgery reduced the risk of recurrence or metastasis by four-fold during a 2.5 to 4 year follow up period [103]. In prostate cancer, 4 retrospective studies have been done. Biki et al. found a benefit effect of regional anesthesia/analgesia in patients with prostate cancer who underwent surgery with thoracic epidural plus general anesthesia with a 57% lower risk of recurrence compared with general anesthesia plus opioids [104]. In 2010, Wuethrich et al., suggested that in patient with prostate cancer and general anesthesia combined with epidural analgesia result in improved clinical progression- free survival and reduced risk of cancer progression [105]. This contrast with Tsui et al., who performed a secondary analysis on patient undergoing radical prostatectomy [106]. Patients were randomized to receive either general anesthesia alone or combined general/epidural anesthesia. No difference was observed between the control and epidural group in disease free survival. These findings are supported by Forget et al., who also did not found association between epidural analgesia and biochemical recurrence rate [107]. In 2013, a retrospective study by Wuethrich et al., suggested that general anesthesia combined with epidural analgesia did not reduce the risk of cancer progression or improve survival after radical prostatectomy [108]. In the case of colon cancer the result are not promising. Cummings and colleagues did not find a positive correlation between the use of epidural anesthesia and colon cancer surgery [109]. In addition Myles et al., concluded that cancer recurrence rate and mortality are similar in patients who undergo surgery with either with general anesthesia combined with epidural anesthesia/analgesia or general anesthesia with opioid analgesia in major abdominal surgery [110, 111]. In ovarian cancer, Oliveira and colleagues, suggested that the intraoperative used of epidural anesthesia reduces the risk of cancer recurrence [112]. In a recent study published by our group, we were also not able to demonstrate an association between the use of regional analgesia for thoracotomy and non-small cell lung cancer recurrence [113]. Large randomized multicenter clinical trials on melanoma (NCT01588847), breast (NCT00418457), lung (NCT01179308) and colon (NCT00684229) cancers are being conducted and will help to clarify the real benefit of regional anesthesia on cancer recurrence.

In conclusion, surgery stress response can potentially promotes growth of dormant tumor and cancer metastasis process through the shedding of malignant cells, release of pro angiogenic factors, growth factors, catecholamines and prostaglandins. Prostaglandin and catecholamines are key mediators of the potential harmful effect of surgery on cancer recurrence and metastasis. These molecules can act either directly on tumor cells and immune cells or indirectly by altering the tumor microenvironment. As a consequence these molecules produces an immune disarrangement which include a complex interaction between the endocrine, metabolic and immunological system that will results in activation of the HPA axis, inflammation, NK cells suppression and shift towards a Th2 response, which consequently translate to immune suppression. The observation that the excess of PGs and catecholamines during the perioperative period in cancer patients may increase the risk of metastasis and cancer recurrence has developed a new window of opportunity to intervene and perhaps contribute to a better long-term outcome.

References

[1]   Giannoudis, P.V., et al., Surgical stress response. *Injury*, 2006. 37 Suppl 5: p. S3-9.

[2]   Brotman, D.J., S.H. Golden, and I.S. Wittstein, The cardiovascular toll of stress. *Lancet*, 2007. 370(9592): p. 1089-100.

[3] SELYE, H., Stress and the general adaptation syndrome. *Br Med J*, 1950. 1(4667): p. 1383-92.

[4] McEwen, B.S., Stressed or stressed out: what is the difference? *J Psychiatry Neurosci*, 2005. 30(5): p. 315-8.

[5] Millan, M.J., The induction of pain: an integrative review. *Prog Neurobiol*, 1999. 57(1): p. 1-164.

[6] Renn, C.L. and S.G. Dorsey, The physiology and processing of pain: a review. *AACN Clin Issues*, 2005. 16(3): p. 277-90; quiz 413-5.

[7] Eisenhofer, G., I.J. Kopin, and D.S. Goldstein, Catecholamine metabolism: a contemporary view with implications for physiology and medicine. *Pharmacol Rev*, 2004. 56(3): p. 331-49.

[8] KOPIN, I.J. and E.K. GORDON, Metabolism of norepinephrine-H3 released by tyramine and reserpine. *J Pharmacol Exp Ther*, 1962. 138: p. 351-9.

[9] Ogawa, K., et al., Suppression of cellular immunity by surgical stress. *Surgery*, 2000. 127(3): p. 329-36.

[10] Kadoi, Y., Blood glucose control in the perioperative period. *Minerva Anestesiol*, 2012. 78(5): p. 574-95.

[11] Kushner, I., The phenomenon of the acute phase response. *Ann N Y Acad Sci*, 1982. 389: p. 39-48.

[12] Cuesta, J.M. and M. Singer, The stress response and critical illness: a review. *Crit Care Med*, 2012. 40(12): p. 3283-9.

[13] Finnerty, C.C., et al., The surgically induced stress response. *JPEN J Parenter Enteral Nutr*, 2013. 37(5 Suppl): p. 21S-9S.

[14] Desborough, J.P., The stress response to trauma and surgery. Br *J Anaesth*, 2000. 85(1): p. 109-17.

[15] Jameson, P., et al., The effect of cortisol suppression on interleukin-6 and white blood cell responses to surgery. *Acta Anaesthesiol Scand*, 1997. 41(2): p. 304-8.

[16] Ricciotti, E. and G.A. FitzGerald, Prostaglandins and inflammation. *Arterioscler Thromb Vasc Biol*, 2011. 31(5): p. 986-1000.

[17] Wang, Z.Q., et al., A newly identified role for superoxide in inflammatory pain. *J Pharmacol Exp Ther*, 2004. 309(3): p. 869-78.

[18] Silva, R.O., et al., Phytol, a diterpene alcohol, inhibits the inflammatory response by reducing cytokine production and oxidative stress. *Fundam Clin Pharmacol*, 2013.

[19] Sheeran, P. and G.M. Hall, Cytokines in anaesthesia. *Br J Anaesth*, 1997. 78(2): p. 201-19.

[20] Netea, M.G., B.J. Kullberg, and J.W. Van der Meer, Circulating cytokines as mediators of fever. *Clin Infect Dis,* 2000. 31 Suppl 5: p. S178-84.

[21] Kemik, O., et al., The relationship among acute-phase response proteins, cytokines and hormones in cachectic patients with colon cancer. *World J Surg Oncol,* 2010. 8: p. 85.

[22] Bartal, I., et al., Immune perturbations in patients along the perioperative period: alterations in cell surface markers and leukocyte subtypes before and after surgery. *Brain Behav Immun,* 2010. 24(3): p. 376-86.

[23] Dinarello, C.A., et al., Tumor necrosis factor (cachectin) is an endogenous pyrogen and induces production of interleukin 1. *J Exp Med,* 1986. 163(6): p. 1433-50.

[24] Dinarello, C.A., et al., Interleukin-6 as an endogenous pyrogen: induction of prostaglandin E2 in brain but not in peripheral blood mononuclear cells. *Brain Res,* 1991. 562(2): p. 199-206.

[25] Dinarello, C.A., Infection, fever, and exogenous and endogenous pyrogens: some concepts have changed. *J Endotoxin Res,* 2004. 10(4): p. 201-22.

[26] Reinold, H., et al., Spinal inflammatory hyperalgesia is mediated by prostaglandin E receptors of the EP2 subtype. *J Clin Invest,* 2005. 115(3): p. 673-9.

[27] Goto, S., et al., Analysis of Th1 and Th2 cytokine production by peripheral blood mononuclear cells as a parameter of immunological dysfunction in advanced cancer patients. *Cancer Immunol Immunother,* 1999. 48(8): p. 435-42.

[28] Jiang, J., C. Wu, and B. Lu, Cytokine-induced killer cells promote antitumor immunity. *J Transl Med,* 2013. 11: p. 83.

[29] Decker, D., et al., Surgical stress induces a shift in the type-1/type-2 T-helper cell balance, suggesting down-regulation of cell-mediated and up-regulation of antibody-mediated immunity commensurate to the trauma. *Surgery,* 1996. 119(3): p. 316-25.

[30] Ishikawa, M., et al., Perioperative immune responses in cancer patients undergoing digestive surgeries. *World J Surg Oncol,* 2009. 7: p. 7.

[31] Boumpas, D.T., et al., Glucocorticoid therapy for immune-mediated diseases: basic and clinical correlates. *Ann Intern Med,* 1993. 119(12): p. 1198-208.

[32] Huang, M., et al., Human non-small cell lung cancer cells express a type 2 cytokine pattern. *Cancer Res,* 1995. 55(17): p. 3847-53.

[33] Monjan, A.A. and M.I. Collector, Stress-induced modulation of the immune response. *Science*, 1977. 196(4287): p. 307-8.

[34] Bozza, F.A., et al., Cytokine profiles as markers of disease severity in sepsis: a multiplex analysis. *Crit Care*, 2007. 11(2): p. R49.

[35] Riedemann, N.C., R.F. Guo, and P.A. Ward, The enigma of sepsis. *J Clin Invest*, 2003. 112(4): p. 460-7.

[36] Juan P. Cata, V.G., Daniel I. Sessler *How regional analgesia might reduce postoperative cancer recurrence.* 2011. Volume 5, 345–355.

[37] Guller, U., et al., Disseminated single tumor cells as detected by real-time quantitative polymerase chain reaction represent a prognostic factor in patients undergoing surgery for colorectal cancer. *Ann Surg*, 2002. 236(6): p. 768-75; discussion 775-6.

[38] Yamashita, J.I., et al., Detection of circulating tumor cells in patients with non-small cell lung cancer undergoing lobectomy by video-assisted thoracic surgery: a potential hazard for intraoperative hematogenous tumor cell dissemination. *J Thorac Cardiovasc Surg*, 2000. 119(5): p. 899-905.

[39] Schmidt, B., et al., Detection of circulating prostate cells during radical prostatectomy by standardized PSMA RT-PCR: association with positive lymph nodes and high malignant grade. *Anticancer Res*, 2003. 23(5A): p. 3991-9.

[40] O'Byrne, K.J., et al., Vascular endothelial growth factor, platelet-derived endothelial cell growth factor and angiogenesis in non-small-cell lung cancer. *Br J Cancer*, 2000. 82(8): p. 1427-32.

[41] Hogan, B.V., et al., Surgery induced immunosuppression. *Surgeon*, 2011. 9(1): p. 38-43.

[42] Lejeune, F.J., Is surgical trauma prometastatic? *Anticancer Res*, 2012. 32(3): p. 947-51.

[43] Cardinale, F., et al., Perioperative period: immunological modifications. *Int J Immunopathol Pharmacol*, 2011. 24(3 Suppl): p. S3-12.

[44] Greenfeld, K., et al., Immune suppression while awaiting surgery and following it: dissociations between plasma cytokine levels, their induced production, and NK cell cytotoxicity. *Brain Behav Immun*, 2007. 21(4): p. 503-13.

[45] Melamed, R., et al., Suppression of natural killer cell activity and promotion of tumor metastasis by ketamine, thiopental, and halothane, but not by propofol: mediating mechanisms and prophylactic measures. *Anesth Analg*, 2003. 97(5): p. 1331-9.

[46] Kurosawa, S. and M. Kato, Anesthetics, immune cells, and immune responses. *J Anesth,* 2008. 22(3): p. 263-77.

[47] Vallejo, R., et al., Perioperative immunosuppression in cancer patients. *J Environ Pathol Toxicol Oncol,* 2003. 22(2): p. 139-46.

[48] Antoni, M.H., et al., The influence of bio-behavioural factors on tumour biology: pathways and mechanisms. *Nat Rev Cancer,* 2006. 6(3): p. 240-8.

[49] Bernabé, D.G., et al., Stress hormones increase cell proliferation and regulates interleukin-6 secretion in human oral squamous cell carcinoma cells. *Brain Behav Immun,* 2011. 25(3): p. 574-83.

[50] Thaker, P.H., et al., Chronic stress promotes tumor growth and angiogenesis in a mouse model of ovarian carcinoma. *Nat Med,* 2006. 12(8): p. 939-44.

[51] Landen, C.N., et al., Neuroendocrine modulation of signal transducer and activator of transcription-3 in ovarian cancer. *Cancer Res,* 2007. 67(21): p. 10389-96.

[52] Bookout, A.L., et al., Targeting Gbetagamma signaling to inhibit prostate tumor formation and growth. *J Biol Chem,* 2003. 278(39): p. 37569-73.

[53] Sastry, K.S., et al., Epinephrine protects cancer cells from apoptosis via activation of cAMP-dependent protein kinase and BAD phosphorylation. *J Biol Chem,* 2007. 282(19): p. 14094-100.

[54] Hellstrand, K. and S. Hermodsson, An immunopharmacological analysis of adrenaline-induced suppression of human natural killer cell cytotoxicity. *Int Arch Allergy Appl Immunol,* 1989. 89(4): p. 334-41.

[55] Inbar, S., et al., Do stress responses promote leukemia progression? An animal study suggesting a role for epinephrine and prostaglandin-E2 through reduced NK activity. *PLoS One,* 2011. 6(4): p. e19246.

[56] Shakhar, G. and S. Ben-Eliyahu, In vivo beta-adrenergic stimulation suppresses natural killer activity and compromises resistance to tumor metastasis in rats. *J Immunol,* 1998. 160(7): p. 3251-8.

[57] Elenkov, I.J., et al., Modulatory effects of glucocorticoids and catecholamines on human interleukin-12 and interleukin-10 production: clinical implications. *Proc Assoc Am Physicians,* 1996. 108(5): p. 374-81.

[58] Benish, M., et al., Perioperative use of beta-blockers and COX-2 inhibitors may improve immune competence and reduce the risk of tumor metastasis. *Ann Surg Oncol,* 2008. 15(7): p. 2042-52.

[59] Melhem-Bertrandt, A., et al., Beta-blocker use is associated with improved relapse-free survival in patients with triple-negative breast cancer. *J Clin Oncol*, 2011. 29(19): p. 2645-52.

[60] Aydiner, A., et al., Does Beta-blocker Therapy Improve the Survival of Patients with Metastatic Non-small Cell Lung Cancer? *Asian Pac J Cancer Prev*, 2013. 14(10): p. 6109-14.

[61] Vitale, C., et al., The corticosteroid-induced inhibitory effect on NK cell function reflects down-regulation and/or dysfunction of triggering receptors involved in natural cytotoxicity. *Eur J Immunol*, 2004. 34(11): p. 3028-38.

[62] Shakhar, G. and B. Blumenfeld, Glucocorticoid involvement in suppression of NK activity following surgery in rats. *J Neuroimmunol*, 2003. 138(1-2): p. 83-91.

[63] Komori, K., et al., Cytokine patterns and the effects of a preoperative steroid treatment in the patients with abdominal aortic aneurysms. *Int Angiol*, 1999. 18(3): p. 193-7.

[64] Vecht, C.J., et al., Dose-effect relationship of dexamethasone on Karnofsky performance in metastatic brain tumors: a randomized study of doses of 4, 8, and 16 mg per day. *Neurology*, 1994. 44(4): p. 675-80.

[65] Dietrich, J., et al., Corticosteroids in brain cancer patients: benefits and pitfalls. *Expert Rev Clin Pharmacol*, 2011. 4(2): p. 233-42.

[66] Vyvey, M., Steroids as pain relief adjuvants. *Can Fam Physician*, 2010. 56(12): p. 1295-7, e415.

[67] Riechelmann, R.P., et al., Symptom and medication profiles among cancer patients attending a palliative care clinic. *Support Care Cancer*, 2007. 15(12): p. 1407-12.

[68] Egberts, J.H., et al., Dexamethasone reduces tumor recurrence and metastasis after pancreatic tumor resection in SCID mice. *Cancer Biol Ther*, 2008. 7(7): p. 1044-50.

[69] Holbrook, N.J., W.I. Cox, and H.C. Horner, Direct suppression of natural killer activity in human peripheral blood leukocyte cultures by glucocorticoids and its modulation by interferon. *Cancer Res*, 1983. 43(9): p. 4019-25.

[70] Bush, K.A., et al., Glucocorticoid receptor mediated suppression of natural killer cell activity: identification of associated deacetylase and corepressor molecules. *Cell Immunol*, 2012. 275(1-2): p. 80-9.

[71] De Oliveira, G.S., et al., Is Dexamethasone Associated with Recurrence of Ovarian Cancer? *Anesth Analg*, 2013.

[72] Szumiło, J., et al., *[Cyclooxygenase inhibitors in chemoprevention and treatment of esophageal squamous cell carcinoma]*. Pol Merkur Lekarski, 2009. 27(161): p. 408-12.

[73] Gurpinar, E., W.E. Grizzle, and G.A. Piazza, COX-Independent Mechanisms of Cancer Chemoprevention by Anti-Inflammatory Drugs. *Front Oncol*, 2013. 3: p. 181.

[74] Chan, T.A., Nonsteroidal anti-inflammatory drugs, apoptosis, and colon-cancer chemoprevention. *Lancet Oncol*, 2002. 3(3): p. 166-74.

[75] Wang, D. and R.N. Dubois, Prostaglandins and cancer. *Gut*, 2006. 55(1): p. 115-22.

[76] Martinet, L., et al., PGE2 inhibits natural killer and gamma delta T cell cytotoxicity triggered by NKR and TCR through a cAMP-mediated PKA type I-dependent signaling. *Biochem Pharmacol*, 2010. 80(6): p. 838-45.

[77] Chattopadhyay, S., et al., Tumor-shed PGE(2) impairs IL2Rgammac-signaling to inhibit CD4 T cell survival: regulation by theaflavins. *PLoS One*, 2009. 4(10): p. e7382.

[78] Ahmadi, M., D.C. Emery, and D.J. Morgan, Prevention of both direct and cross-priming of antitumor CD8+ T-cell responses following overproduction of prostaglandin E2 by tumor cells in vivo. *Cancer Res*, 2008. 68(18): p. 7520-9.

[79] Maekawa, M., et al., Increased expression of cyclooxygenase-2 to -1 in human colorectal cancers and adenomas, but not in hyperplastic polyps. *Jpn J Clin Oncol*, 1998. 28(7): p. 421-6.

[80] Gupta, S., et al., Over-expression of cyclooxygenase-2 in human prostate adenocarcinoma. *Prostate*, 2000. 42(1): p. 73-8.

[81] Parrett, M., et al., Cyclooxygenase-2 gene expression in human breast cancer. *Int J Oncol*, 1997. 10(3): p. 503-7.

[82] Hu, M., et al., Role of COX-2 in epithelial-stromal cell interactions and progression of ductal carcinoma in situ of the breast. *Proc Natl Acad Sci U S A*, 2009. 106(9): p. 3372-7.

[83] Rolland, P.H., et al., Prostaglandin in human breast cancer: Evidence suggesting that an elevated prostaglandin production is a marker of high metastatic potential for neoplastic cells. *J Natl Cancer Inst*, 1980. 64(5): p. 1061-70.

[84] Eberhart, C.E., et al., Up-regulation of cyclooxygenase 2 gene expression in human colorectal adenomas and adenocarcinomas. *Gastroenterology*, 1994. 107(4): p. 1183-8.

[85]   Shiff, S.J. and B. Rigas, Nonsteroidal anti-inflammatory drugs and colorectal cancer: evolving concepts of their chemopreventive actions. *Gastroenterology*, 1997. 113(6): p. 1992-8.

[86]   Masferrer, J.L., et al., Antiangiogenic and antitumor activities of cyclooxygenase-2 inhibitors. *Cancer Res*, 2000. 60(5): p. 1306-11.

[87]   Harris, R.E., et al., Chemoprevention of breast cancer in rats by celecoxib, a cyclooxygenase 2 inhibitor. *Cancer Res*, 2000. 60(8): p. 2101-3.

[88]   Schreinemachers, D.M. and R.B. Everson, Aspirin use and lung, colon, and breast cancer incidence in a prospective study. *Epidemiology*, 1994. 5(2): p. 138-46.

[89]   Harris, R.E., J. Beebe-Donk, and H.M. Schuller, Chemoprevention of lung cancer by non-steroidal anti-inflammatory drugs among cigarette smokers. *Oncol Rep*, 2002. 9(4): p. 693-5.

[90]   Muscat, J.E., et al., Risk of lung carcinoma among users of nonsteroidal antiinflammatory drugs. *Cancer*, 2003. 97(7): p. 1732-6.

[91]   Ratliff, T.L., Aspirin, ibuprofen, and other non-steroidal anti-inflammatory drugs in cancer prevention: a critical review of non-selective COX-2 blockade (review). *J Urol*, 2005. 174(2): p. 787-8.

[92]   Liu, J.F., et al., A preliminary study on the postoperative survival of patients given aspirin after resection for squamous cell carcinoma of the esophagus or adenocarcinoma of the cardia. *Ann Surg Oncol*, 2009. 16(5): p. 1397-402.

[93]   Martin, L.A., et al., Pre-surgical study of the biological effects of the selective cyclo-oxygenase-2 inhibitor celecoxib in patients with primary breast cancer. *Breast Cancer Res Treat*, 2010. 123(3): p. 829-36.

[94]   Sooriakumaran, P., et al., A randomized controlled trial investigating the effects of celecoxib in patients with localized prostate cancer. *Anticancer Res*, 2009. 29(5): p. 1483-8.

[95]   Beilin, B., et al., Low-dose ketamine affects immune responses in humans during the early postoperative period. *Br J Anaesth*, 2007. 99(4): p. 522-7.

[96]   Schneemilch, C.E., T. Schilling, and U. Bank, Effects of general anaesthesia on inflammation. *Best Pract Res Clin Anaesthesiol*, 2004. 18(3): p. 493-507.

[97]   Matsuoka, H., et al., Inhalation anesthetics induce apoptosis in normal peripheral lymphocytes in vitro. *Anesthesiology*, 2001. 95(6): p. 1467-72.

[98] Gupta, K., et al., Morphine stimulates angiogenesis by activating proangiogenic and survival-promoting signaling and promotes breast tumor growth. *Cancer Res,* 2002. 62(15): p. 4491-8.

[99] Lazarczyk, M., E. Matyja, and A.W. Lipkowski, A comparative study of morphine stimulation and biphalin inhibition of human glioblastoma T98G cell proliferation in vitro. *Peptides,* 2010. 31(8): p. 1606-12.

[100] Greeneltch, K.M., et al., Chronic morphine treatment promotes specific Th2 cytokine production by murine T cells in vitro via a Fas/Fas ligand-dependent mechanism. *J Immunol,* 2005. 175(8): p. 4999-5005.

[101] Roy, S., et al., Morphine directs T cells toward T(H2) differentiation. *Surgery,* 2001. 130(2): p. 304-9.

[102] Koltun, W.A., et al., Awake epidural anesthesia is associated with improved natural killer cell cytotoxicity and a reduced stress response. *Am J Surg,*

[103] Exadaktylos, A.K., et al., Can anesthetic technique for primary breast cancer surgery affect recurrence or metastasis? *Anesthesiology,* 2006. 105(4): p. 660-4.

[104] Biki, B., et al., Anesthetic technique for radical prostatectomy surgery affects cancer recurrence: a retrospective analysis. *Anesthesiology,* 2008. 109(2): p. 180-7.

[105] Wuethrich, P.Y., et al., Potential influence of the anesthetic technique used during open radical prostatectomy on prostate cancer-related outcome: a retrospective study. *Anesthesiology,* 2010. 113(3): p. 570-6.

[106] Tsui, B.C., et al., Epidural anesthesia and cancer recurrence rates after radical prostatectomy. *Can J Anaesth,* 2010. 57(2): p. 107-12.

[107] Forget, P., et al., Do intraoperative analgesics influence oncological outcomes after radical prostatectomy for prostate cancer? *Eur J Anaesthesiol,* 2011. 28(12): p. 830-5.

[108] Wuethrich, P.Y., et al., Epidural analgesia during open radical prostatectomy does not improve long-term cancer-related outcome: a retrospective study in patients with advanced prostate cancer. *PLoS One,* 2013. 8(8): p. e72873.

[109] Cummings, K.C., et al., A comparison of epidural analgesia and traditional pain management effects on survival and cancer recurrence after colectomy: a population-based study. *Anesthesiology,* 2012. 116(4): p. 797-806.

[110] Gottschalk, A., et al., Review article: the role of the perioperative period in recurrence after cancer surgery. *Anesth Analg,* 2010. 110(6): p. 1636-43.

[111] Myles, P.S., et al., Perioperative epidural analgesia for major abdominal surgery for cancer and recurrence-free survival: randomised trial. *BMJ*, 2011. 342: p. d1491.

[112] de Oliveira, G.S., et al., Intraoperative neuraxial anesthesia but not postoperative neuraxial analgesia is associated with increased relapse-free survival in ovarian cancer patients after primary cytoreductive surgery. *Reg Anesth Pain Med*, 2011. 36(3): p. 271-7.

[113] Cata, J.P., et al., Effects of postoperative epidural analgesia on recurrence-free and overall survival in patients with nonsmall cell lung cancer. *J Clin Anesth*, 2013.

In: General and Abdominal Surgery
Editor: Kassandra Sarah Slavomir

ISBN: 978-1-63117-440-7
© 2014 Nova Science Publishers, Inc.

Chapter 5

Perioperative Blood Transfusions and Its Complications

Hao Wang and Juan P. Cata
Department of Anesthesiology and Perioperative Medicine,
University of Texas MD Anderson Cancer Center,
Houston, TX, US

Abstract

The rate of perioperative blood transfusions is still high. They are commonly given to treat perioperative anemia and improve the delivery of oxygen but unfortunately they can also be associated to several adverse reactions. These can range from mild febrile reactions to anaphylactic shock. Less recognized complications associated to the administration of blood products include transfusion-related acute lung injury, graft-versus-host disease, transfusion-related fluid overload and transfusion-related immune suppression. This particular last complication has been the focus of study of several investigators because of the clinical implications on cancer biology, specifically on cancer recurrence. Perturbations in the Th1/Th2 balance and an impaired innate and adaptive immunity are hallmarks of the so-called transfusion related immune suppression. Although, the results from clinical studies evaluating the effects of transfusion-related immune suppression on oncological outcomes are mixed, a meta-analysis in patients with colorectal cancer suggests the association between blood transfusions and cancer recurrence.

Introduction

The need for blood transfusion in the United States is still very high. According to estimates by the Center for Disease Control (CDC) and the American Red Cross, about every two seconds someone in the U.S. needs blood. On average, approximately more than 4.5 million Americans receive blood each year and the average red blood cell (RBC) transfusion is approximately about 3 pints [1, 2].

Currently, there is no artificial alternative to human blood that exists. Each year, there are approximately 15.7 million blood donations collected in the United States (roughly one pint of blood per donation). The percentage of people that donate in the United State is not very high either; less than 10% of the population actually donates blood per year [2]. Another fact that makes the blood supply scarce is that blood products are perishable; donated RBCs can only last up to 42 days, platelet concentrates lasting less than 5 days, and frozen plasma can last up to one year [3]. Due to the fact that blood is a scarce resource, blood transfusions tend to be very expensive; in the United States a single blood unit costed approximately range from $522 to $1183 in 2010 [4]. A recent study by Shander et al. showed that largely depending on the transfusion rate, the annual expenditure on blood and transfusion related activities, can range from $1.6 million to $6.2 million per hospital [4].

Perioperative blood transfusion is a therapy that is potentially lifesaving in many situations but is still inherently hazardous. The combination of surgery-induced stress, usage of volatile anesthetics and opioids contribute to immune suppression and can be further exaggerated by the administration of blood products. Specifically, cancer surgical patients that undergo perioperative blood transfusions have greater exposure to potential harm [5-8]. There has been an association between perioperative transfusion of allogeneic blood products and risk for recurrence shown in randomized trials in colorectal cancer [9]. Current evidence show that there are many factors that may contribute to the possible recurrence of cancer after perioperative blood transfusion, such as transfusion volume, blood product storage duration, and timing of transfusions [10-13]. Hence, several authors have suggested to develop and mandate patient-specific blood management protocols for the perioperative blood period to decrease the potential need for blood transfusions.

Complications Associated with Blood Transfusions

Although blood transfusions are deemed very safe by the CDC and the chances of having an adverse reaction is considered minor, there are still a good amount of unwanted effects that could possibly occur from administering blood transfusions [1]. Autologous blood transfusions are generally accepted as the safer method that contains less risk and results in fewer post-transfusion complications. Allogeneic blood transfusions pose more risks such as incompatibility, transmission of infectious diseases, and allergic reactions [14]. Importantly, both types of transfusions can cause fluid overload and transfusion-related immune suppression (TRIM) [15]. The most common negative reactions from perioperative blood transfusion are allergic and febrile reactions; they make up for more than half of the reported adverse reactions. Another type of rare but very serious adverse reaction is infection related reactions [14].

Allergic Reactions

Although patients are given blood that matches their specific blood type (ABO group) and Rh type (positive or negative), there is still a possibility that the patient could have allergic reaction to parts of the transfused blood. Allergic reactions are common and usually not very serious. The majority of the allergic reactions from transfusions is caused by the presence of foreign proteins in the donors' plasma and is mostly immunoglobin E (IgE) mediated [16]. Symptoms of allergic reactions are usually limited to pruritus and urticaria. In such cases, transfusions should then be stopped immediately and anti-histamines should be administered for treatment. In rare instances, a more serious allergic reaction may occur and be manifested as respiratory symptoms, hypotension and shock [14].

Febrile Associated Complications

Febrile reactions are noted for the development of fever during or soon after the transfusion. Febrile non-hemolytic transfusion reactions (FNHTR) are the most frequent reaction reported due to transfusions. These reactions are usually not life threatening. FNHTR results from the interaction of donor leucocyte antigen and antibodies present in the patient's plasma. Symptoms of FNHTR are fever and/or chills in the absence of hemolysis during or up to 4 hours after the transfusion. The reactions of FNHTR cases are generally mild, but are dependent upon leucocyte concentration and speed of the transfusion. Antipyretics should be administered for treatment [14].

Infectious Related Complications

Transfusion-transmitted infections (TTI) occur when a bacterium, virus, prion or other potential pathogen is transmitted via donor blood to the patient. TTI cases are very rare due to the fact that donated blood is screened and tested for pathogens before accepted by hospitals. In the cases where bacterial contamination occurs, the potential severe sepsis in the patient is partnered with high mortality rates.

Symptoms include high fever, shivering, erythema and cardiovascular collapse [17]. Viral infections have been greatly reduced since the 1980s due to the fact that donor blood is now screened for Hepatitis B, Hepatitis C, Human Immundeficiency Virus, Syphilis, and human T cell lymphotrophic virus [1]. However, viral infections may still occur if the donor is infectious but screening tests are negative. Viral infections will likely cause the patient to develop the disease of the specific viral pathogen is present in donor blood. The estimated risks of contacting TTI are listed in Table 1.

Table 1. Risk of transfusion-transmitted infection

Disease	Estimated Risk
HIV	1 / 2.3 million
Hepatitis B	1 / 350,000
Hepatitis C	1 / 2 million
Human T-lymphotrophic virus	1 / 2 million
Bacterial infection in blood	1 / 1 million

Source: Center for Disease Control (2010).

Incompatibility Related Complications

Incompatibility between the antibodies in the donor RBC antigens and recipient (patient) plasma antibodies can result in hemolytic transfusion reaction. There are two types of hemolytic transfusion reaction: acute hemolytic transfusion reaction (AHTR) and delayed hemolytic transfusion reaction (DHTR) [18]. The interaction between donor RBC antigens and patient plasma antibodies due to incompatibility will bring about an antigen-antibody complex that causes complement fixation, intravascular hemolysis and elimination of transfused blood [18]. In AHTR, this occurs during, immediately after, or within 24 hours of a transfusion when patient is given incompatible blood type. Symptoms include fever, pain, nausea and kidney failure (in severe cases). The severity of the reaction is correlated with patient's antibody concentration. In AHTR, most of the severe reactions are most frequently the result of ABO incompatibility. In DHTR, incompatibility of minor blood groups such as Rhesus and Kidd is responsible for the antigen-antibody complex. DHTR occurs between 24 to 48 hours after the transfusion takes place. Symptoms of DHTR are usually milder than AHTR and occur at a slower rate. It usually takes one to four weeks to notice a decrease in RBC levels. However, DHTR can be diagnosed with laboratory testing [16, 18].

Other Complications

Transfusion-related acute lung injury (TRALI) is a serious complication that occurs as the result of an increased permeability at the level of the pulmonary vasculature [19]. It usually occurs within one to six hours of transfusion and clinically patients present different degrees of pulmonary edema and subsequent hypoxemia. TRALI is reported to be one of the most common and serious causes of major morbidity and death post transfusion [1, 19].

Transfusion-associated graft versus host disease (TAGVHD) is a very rare complication of blood transfusion that usually occurs in those patients who are already immunocompromised [16, 18]. It occurs when donor T-lymphocytes introduced by the blood transfusion attacks the recipient cells. Symptoms include maculopapular rash, fever, abdominal pain, and abnormal liver function tests. TAGVHD occurs between two days and six weeks after transfusion. Although rare, this inflammatory response is difficult to treat and 90% of the cases are fatal.

Transfusion-Related Immune Modulation and Cancer Recurrence

One of the major drawbacks of perioperative blood transfusion is the fact that it causes transfusion-related immune modulation (TRIM), a condition that negatively affects the human immune system. TRIM is linked to several numbers of complications, including cancer recurrence in cancer patients. TRIM can be caused by several mechanisms such as suppression of cytotoxic cell and monocyte activity, release of immunosuppressive prostaglandins, inhibition of interleukin-2 (IL-2) production, increase in suppressor T-cell activity and a decrease in the function of natural killer (NK) cells [20]. The accumulation of lysophosphatidylcholines and growth factors, released from white blood cells are also involved in transfusion-related immune suppression [21, 22].

In an attempt to reduce the number of bioactive substances, allogeneic blood products are leucoreduced before storage (Figure 1). It is important to note that even though leucocyte numbers are reduced 3 log (99.9) after undergoing leucocyte reduction via screen filters, there are still few leucocyte that may still trigger an abnormal immune response in the recipient [21]. In non-leucoreduced RBC units, there are increased concentrations of Th1 (antitumoral) and predominately Th2 cytokines (pro-turmoral) compared to leucoreduced pRBC units [23-25]. It is also seen that the exposure of leucoreduced stored RBC supernatant reacts to whole blood by inducing regulatory T-cell (Treg) activation. The activation of Treg cells suppresses the functions of Th1 responses by CD4$^+$ and CD8$^+$ T cells [26-28]. This is especially important in cancer patients, as NK cells and cytotoxic T lymphocytes (CTLs) engage in tumor killing and Th1 cells boost cytotoxic immunity, both essential to combating tumor progression. The activation of Treg cells to become immune suppressive is also antigen non-specific. These findings may contribute to the explanation on why inflammation and immunosuppression still occurs after transfusions of stored leucoreduced allogeneic blood.

An important correlation suggested by multiple clinical studies is that the severity of the pro-inflammatory burden caused by perioperative blood transfusion appears to be directly proportional to the storage age of blood products. Koch and colleagues found confounding evidence that the longer RBC products are stored, the less effective and safe it is for use [3].

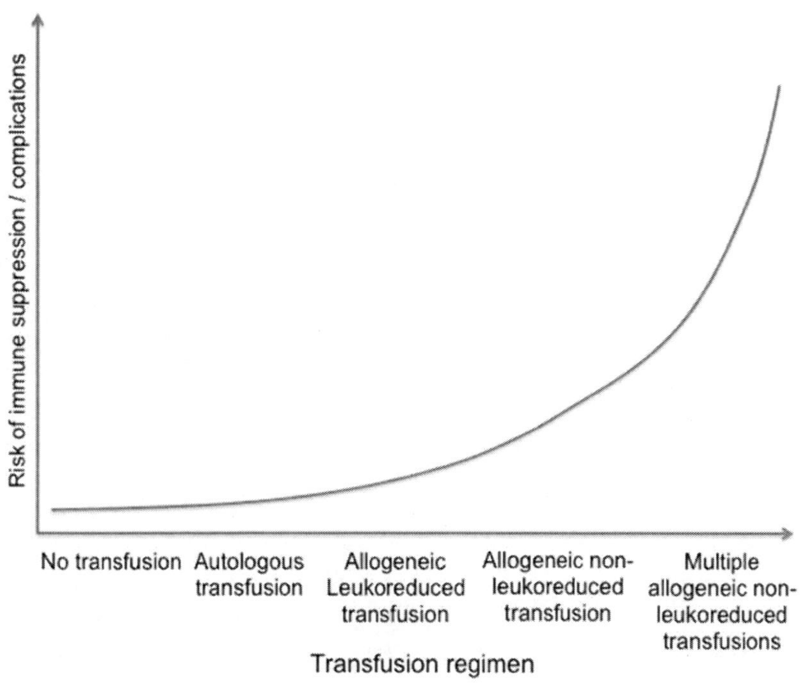

Figure 1. Risk of transfusion-related immune suppression.

Another study by the Kanter group shows that platelet concentrates that are stored for longer than 6 days have a significant higher concentration of oncogenic and angiogenic growth factors [29]. In a recent laboratory study, the evidence has suggested that aged RBCs (older than 9 days) greatly increase the risk of tumor progression in non-immunogenic animals, where as fresh RBCs had no such effects [30].

Packed platelet concentrates also contain bioactive products such as cytokines, chemokines, microparticles, and growth factors that play a major role in transfusion related immune suppression and modulation. The concentration of these bioactive products greatly accumulates after just one hour of transfusion [31]. One of the important bioactive products released via platelet transfusion is the CD40 ligand, a protein known to be able to trigger an inflammatory response in endothelial cells, and leading to the recruitment of leukocytes [32].

Fresh-frozen plasma (FFP) is a blood product free of RBCs, leukocytes, and platelets. It is rich in coagulation factors, such as fibrinogen, Factor V, Factor VIII and with Th$_2$ cytokines [33]. Recent studies have suggested that the perioperative transfusion of FFP has negative impacts in terms of overall survival rate [34]. Patients with colorectal cancer liver metastasis who underwent elective hepatic surgery had a worse prognosis in terms of overall survival rate when given perioperative FFP transfusion. [34] In another study done by the same group, FFP is also found to be associated with poor therapeutic outcome in patients with pancreatic ductal adenocarcinoma who have undergone elective pancreatic resection [35]. A study published in 2008 also showed that perioperative FFP transfusion was associated with increased risk of infection in critically ill surgical patients [36]. Currently, there has not yet been a study on whether perioperative transfusion of FFP is associated with increased risk of cancer recurrence.

There have been multiple clinical studies trying to link perioperative blood transfusion to tumor progression. Early clinical studies in the 90s, mostly retrospective, suggested that there is a positive relationship between allogeneic perioperative blood transfusion and risk of cancer recurrence and mortality after oncological surgery. However, multiple investigators who did not identify an association between blood transfusion and cancer recurrence have disputed these findings [15]. The most significant current evidence comes from a large meta-analysis in colorectal cancer (table 2). The study done by the Cochrane group suggests that there is an increased risk of cancer recurrence in patients with colorectal cancer that received perioperative blood transfusions [9]. This finding is still unclear and less understood in other types of cancers. A recent study from our group failed to show an association between perioperative blood transfusion and recurrence of non-small cell lung cancer [37].

Currently, the benefits of autologous perioperative blood transfusion over allogeneic perioperative blood transfusion in cancer patients are unclear and disputed. An early observational study in head and neck cancer surgery patients suggested that allogeneic blood transfusions, compared to autologous blood transfusions, had a 40% increase in cancer recurrence [38]. However, these results are in conflict with other studies, such as a randomized controlled trial in colorectal cancer patients who underwernt surgical tumor resection and randomized to allogeneic versus autologous blood transfusions and showed no significant difference in risk of cancer recurrence [39]. A study with limited data in patients with hepatic cellular carcinoma shows that the collection and distribution of autologous blood during the perioperative period appears to be safe [40, 41]. Another small retrospective study suggests that patients with hepatoceullar carcinoma given autologous blood via autotransfusion during hepatectomy had a longer long-term cancer free survival rate compared to those who received allogeneic blood [41].

Intraoperative cell salvage techniques are sometimes used in major surgeries for autologous blood collection, however, a major concern is the potential for re-infusion of malignant cells collected from the surgical site. For example, malignant cells have been found in surgical collected and double-filtered blood samples of patients with hepatocellular carcinoma undergoing liver transplantation [42]. In contrast, several recent studies argue that intraoperative cell salvage techniques and autologous blood transfusion show no significant effect on the rate of recurrence in patients undergoing oncological surgery [43-45].

As mentioned earlier, the presence of leucocytes and other bioactive products in allogeneic blood units may be responsible for immunological suppression. Thus, it is possible to speculate that leucoreduced RBCs may induce less immune suppression and could lead to lower rate of cancer recurrence after oncological surgery. However, there is still no significant clinical evidence to support such theory, and the results of both animal and clinical trials are often conflicting. For example, a recent animal study also found that RBCs rather than leucocytes are associated with the cancer-promoting effects of both allogeneic and autologous blood transfusions [30], while 2 randomized controlled trials did not support a decrease in cancer recurrence risks after leucoreduced pRBC transfusions to patients with gastrointestinal cancer [46, 47].

There have also been studies done to associate cancer recurrence with the transfusion volume, blood product storage duration and timing of transfusions. It is shown that there is a greater risk of cancer recurrence in colorectal cancers when larger volumes (more than 3 units) of blood products are administered [10]. Intraoperative administration of more than 3 units has been associated with a relative increased risk of having a shorter survival period after surgery for ampulla of Vater cancer [10, 11]. A recent meta-analysis reports that the risk of cancer recurrence increases by 40%, 69%, and 102% after 1-2, 3-4, and more than 4 units of pRBC transfusion, respectively [9]. The storage duration of transfused blood units has also been considered a factor that may contribute to the deleterious effects of blood transfusions in terms of immunosupression and cancer recurrence. However, clinical studies have offered little evidence to suggest that the increased duration of storage of blood products contributes to increased risk of cancer recurrence. For example, in a randomized controlled trial, Mynster and Nielsen did not find increased risk of cancer recurrence after transfusion of older versus younger stored blood in patients who had colorectal surgery [48]. In a retrospective study, we could not demonstrate an association between the administration of older blood and recurrence after prostate cancer surgery. [49].

The timing of administration of blood products versus the likelihood of cancer recurrence rate has been tested in colorectal cancer. Pre-, intra-, and postoperative blood transfusion increases the likelihood of cancer recurrence by 50, 74, and 36 % respectively in colorectal cancer patients [9]. In a different retrospective study, postoperative blood transfusions to patients who underwent pancreatic surgery for exocrine tumors was linked to higher mortality [13].

Strategies to Reduce Perioperative Blood Transfusions

Increasing evidence exists for potentially negative effects of perioperative blood transfusions in patients and such evidence demands a more conservative and cautionary approach in deciding the actual need for perioperative blood transfusions. A recent study done by Frank et al. shows that there is a still wide variation in the rate of blood transfusion and a frequent use of perioperative blood transfusions for patients who do not necessarily need it [50]. Strategies to reduce perioperative blood transfusion include but are not limited to: establish an effective blood management program to reduce unnecessary transfusions, and use of alternatives to allogeneic blood. Establishing a patient-specific blood management protocol is crucial to reduction of blood transfusions. Such strategy should focus mainly early preoperative recognition and treatment of anemic patients, surgical efforts to minimize perioperative blood loss, strategies to maintain optimal RBC mass and function, and restrictive volume management [51].

Anemia is arguably the most important risk factor for transfusion, having about 30% of surgical patients present preoperatively with anemia and this might be per se an independent factor for cancer recurrence [52]. Preoperative anemia has also been independently associated with increased mortality in patients undergoing non-cardiac surgery [53]. Clinical studies in patients undergoing orthopedic and cardiac surgery have showed that the successful management of preoperative anemia leads to decrease in the number of blood transfusions as well as improved patient outcomes such as complications, length in hospital stay, and mortality [53]. Recent data continue to support the effectiveness of various hematinics, hemostatic agents and devices, as well as intermittent discontinuation of anticoagulant therapy to mitigate the risk factors for transfusion as mentioned above [54]. In selected patients, studies have also shown that physicians can safely wait until hemoglobin levels fall to 7-8 grams per deciliter before transfusing blood products during surgery [50].

Currently, there are no man-made alternatives that are able to substitute human blood. However, there are multiple strategies that may be used in the perioperative period. According to the Circular of Information for the Use of Human Blood and Blood Components, four different hematinics are identified and should be considered instead of blood transfusion whenever possible and appropriate: iron, folate, vitamin B_{12} and erythropoietin [55]. Spahn and colleagues also suggested that more targeted treatments, such as prothrombin concentrates or fibrinogen concentrates, should be used in order to address associated coagulopathies, and such treatments may be of more value in specific patient settings [53]. The risk-benefit profiles of alternatives to blood transfusion such as hemostatic agents, erythropoiesis-stimulating agents, are still under investigation. The roles of alternatives to blood still need to be better defined by patient-specific treatment plans based on anticipated perioperative blood loss, presence of perioperative anemia, type of surgical procedure, likelihood of blood transfusion and likelihood of coagulopathy. Lastly, quality indicators measuring patient outcomes such as length of hospital stay and mortality need to be incorporated so that alternative to blood transfusions can be more effectively assessed under clinical settings.

Conclusion

Blood transfusion is a still widely used technique to replace blood or blood components lost during surgery, injury or disease. Although can be life-saving, blood transfusions are inherently hazardous and should be only used when the benefits outweighs the risks. Risks of blood transfusion include but are not limited to incompatibility, transmission of infectious diseases, and allergic reactions. Perioperative blood transfusion contains significant risks and is known to cause transfusion-related immune modulation (TRIM) that suppresses the human immune system functions. The combination of surgery-induced stress and usage of anesthetics contribute to immunosuppression and can be further exaggerated by the administration of blood products that create inflammatory burden and immune modulation. Specifically, cancer surgical patients that undergo perioperative blood transfusions have greater exposure to potential harm. Perhaps the best evidence of the association between perioperative transfusion of allogeneic blood products and risk for recurrence is shown in randomized trials studies in colorectal cancer. Currently, both animal and human clinical studies show that there many factors that may contribute to the possible recurrence of cancer after perioperative blood transfusion, such as transfusion volume, blood product storage duration, and timing of transfusions. Due to negative and deleterious effects that come with perioperative blood transfusion, it is desirable to develop a patient-specific blood management protocols for the perioperative period to conserve blood loss and reduce the number and volume of perioperative blood transfusions. Furthermore, alternatives to blood transfusion exist but have yet to have established risk-benefit profiles. The inherent risks of blood transfusion, scarcity of blood, and the increasing cost of blood transfusion should further drive the development of alternatives to blood transfusions in the future.

References

[1] Services USDoHaH: National Blood Collection and Utilization Survey (NBCUS). In.; 2007.

[2] Blood Facts and Statics: Learn About Blood [http://www.redcrossblood .org/learn-about-blood/blood-facts-and-statistics]

[3] Koch CG, Figueroa PI, Li L, Sabik JF, 3rd, Mihaljevic T, Blackstone EH: Red blood cell storage: how long is too long? *The Annals of thoracic surgery* 2013, 96(5):1894-1899.

[4] Shander A, Hofmann A, Ozawa S, Theusinger OM, Gombotz H, Spahn DR: Activity-based costs of blood transfusions in surgical patients at four hospitals. *Transfusion* 2010, 50(4):753-765.

[5] Shiba H, Ishida Y, Wakiyama S, Iida T, Matsumoto M, Sakamoto T, Ito R, Gocho T, Furukawa K, Fujiwara Y *et al*: Negative impact of blood transfusion on recurrence and prognosis of hepatocellular carcinoma after hepatic resection. *Journal of gastrointestinal surgery : official journal of the Society for Surgery of the Alimentary Tract* 2009, 13(9):1636-1642.

[6] Mynster T, Christensen IJ, Moesgaard F, Nielsen HJ: Effects of the combination of blood transfusion and postoperative infectious complications on prognosis after surgery for colorectal cancer. Danish RANX05 Colorectal Cancer Study Group. *The British journal of surgery* 2000, 87(11):1553-1562.

[7]   Nagai S, Fujii T, Kodera Y, Kanda M, Sahin TT, Kanzaki A, Yamada S, Sugimoto H, Nomoto S, Takeda S *et al*: Impact of operative blood loss on survival in invasive ductal adenocarcinoma of the pancreas. *Pancreas* 2011, 40(1):3-9.

[8]   Miki C, Hiro J, Ojima E, Inoue Y, Mohri Y, Kusunoki M: Perioperative allogeneic blood transfusion, the related cytokine response and long-term survival after potentially curative resection of colorectal cancer. *Clinical oncology* 2006, 18(1):60-66.

[9]   Amato A, Pescatori M: Perioperative blood transfusions for the recurrence of colorectal cancer. *The Cochrane database of systematic reviews* 2006(1):CD005033.

[10]   Yao HS, Wang Q, Wang WJ, Hu ZQ: Intraoperative allogeneic red blood cell transfusion in ampullary cancer outcome after curative pancreatoduodenectomy: a clinical study and meta-analysis. *World journal of surgery* 2008, 32(9):2038-2046.

[11]   Zdravkovic D, Bilanovic D, Randjelovic T, Granic M, Djukanovic B, Ivanovic N, Dikic S, Nikolic D, Zdravkovic M, Soldatovic I: Allogeneic blood transfusion in patients in Dukes B stage of colorectal cancer. *Medical oncology* 2011, 28(1):170-174.

[12]   Eickhoff JH, Gote H, Baeck J: Peri-operative blood transfusion in relation to tumour recurrence and death after surgery for prostatic cancer. *British journal of urology* 1991, 68(6):608-611.

[13]   Yeh JJ, Gonen M, Tomlinson JS, Idrees K, Brennan MF, Fong Y: Effect of blood transfusion on outcome after pancreaticoduodenectomy for exocrine tumour of the pancreas. *The British journal of surgery* 2007, 94(4):466-472.

[14]   Maxwell M WM: Complications of blood transfusion. *Continuing Education in Anaesthesia, Critical Care & Pain* 2006, 6(6):225-229.

[15]   Cata JP, Wang H, Gottumukkala V, Reuben J, Sessler DI: Inflammatory response, immunosuppression, and cancer recurrence after perioperative blood transfusions. *British journal of anaesthesia* 2013, 110(5):690-701.

[16]   RD M: Transfusion Therapy. Philadelphia, PA: Churchill Livingstone; 2000.

[17]   Kopko PM, Holland PV: Mechanisms of severe transfusion reactions. *Transfusion clinique et biologique : journal de la Societe francaise de transfusion sanguine* 2001, 8(3):278-281.

[18]   Perrotta PL SE: Blood Transfusion. Oxford: Oxford University Press; 2003.

[19] Bux J: Transfusion-related acute lung injury (TRALI): a serious adverse event of blood transfusion. *Vox sanguinis* 2005, 89(1):1-10.

[20] Vamvakas EC: Possible mechanisms of allogeneic blood transfusion-associated postoperative infection. *Transfusion medicine reviews* 2002, 16(2):144-160.

[21] Blajchman MA: Immunomodulation and blood transfusion. *American journal of therapeutics* 2002, 9(5):389-395.

[22] Ghio M, Contini P, Negrini S, Mazzei C, Zocchi MR, Poggi A: Down regulation of human natural killer cell-mediated cytolysis induced by blood transfusion: role of transforming growth factor-beta(1), soluble Fas ligand, and soluble Class I human leukocyte antigen. *Transfusion* 2011, 51(7):1567-1573.

[23] Weisbach V, Wanke C, Zingsem J, Zimmermann R, Eckstein R: Cytokine generation in whole blood, leukocyte-depleted and temporarily warmed red blood cell concentrates. *Vox sanguinis* 1999, 76(2):100-106.

[24] Stack G, Baril L, Napychank P, Snyder EL: Cytokine generation in stored, white cell-reduced, and bacterially contaminated units of red cells. *Transfusion* 1995, 35(3):199-203.

[25] Shanwell A, Kristiansson M, Remberger M, Ringden O: Generation of cytokines in red cell concentrates during storage is prevented by prestorage white cell reduction. *Transfusion* 1997, 37(7):678-684.

[26] Baecher-Allan C, Brown JA, Freeman GJ, Hafler DA: CD4+CD25high regulatory cells in human peripheral blood. *Journal of immunology* 2001, 167(3):1245-1253.

[27] Piccirillo CA, Shevach EM: Cutting edge: control of CD8+ T cell activation by CD4+CD25+ immunoregulatory cells. *Journal of immunology* 2001, 167(3):1137-1140.

[28] Thornton AM, Shevach EM: Suppressor effector function of CD4+CD25+ immunoregulatory T cells is antigen nonspecific. *Journal of immunology* 2000, 164(1):183-190.

[29] Kanter J, Khan SY, Kelher M, Gore L, Silliman CC: Oncogenic and angiogenic growth factors accumulate during routine storage of apheresis platelet concentrates. *Clinical cancer research : an official journal of the American Association for Cancer Research* 2008, 14(12):3942-3947.

[30] Atzil S, Arad M, Glasner A, Abiri N, Avraham R, Greenfeld K, Rosenne E, Beilin B, Ben-Eliyahu S: Blood transfusion promotes cancer progression: a critical role for aged erythrocytes. *Anesthesiology* 2008, 109(6):989-997.

[31] Apelseth TO, Hervig T, Wentzel-Larsen T, Petersen K, Reikvam H, Bruserud O: A prospective observational study of the effect of platelet transfusions on levels of platelet-derived cytokines, chemokines and interleukins in acute leukaemia patients with severe chemotherapy-induced cytopenia. *European cytokine network* 2011, 22(1):52-62.

[32] Henn V, Slupsky JR, Grafe M, Anagnostopoulos I, Forster R, Muller-Berghaus G, Kroczek RA: CD40 ligand on activated platelets triggers an inflammatory reaction of endothelial cells. *Nature* 1998, 391(6667):591-594.

[33] Theusinger OM, Baulig W, Seifert B, Emmert MY, Spahn DR, Asmis LM: Relative concentrations of haemostatic factors and cytokines in solvent/detergent-treated and fresh-frozen plasma. *British journal of anaesthesia* 2011, 106(4):505-511.

[34] Shiba H, Ishida Y, Haruki K, Furukawa K, Fujiwara Y, Iwase R, Ohkuma M, Ogawa M, Misawa T, Yanaga K: Negative impact of fresh-frozen plasma transfusion on prognosis after hepatic resection for liver metastases from colorectal cancer. *Anticancer research* 2013, 33(6):2723-2728.

[35] Shiba H, Misawa T, Fujiwara Y, Futagawa Y, Furukawa K, Haruki K, Iida T, Iwase R, Yanaga K: Negative impact of fresh-frozen plasma transfusion on prognosis of pancreatic ductal adenocarcinoma after pancreatic resection. *Anticancer research* 2013, 33(9):4041-4047.

[36] Sarani B, Dunkman WJ, Dean L, Sonnad S, Rohrbach JI, Gracias VH: Transfusion of fresh frozen plasma in critically ill surgical patients is associated with an increased risk of infection. *Critical care medicine* 2008, 36(4):1114-1118.

[37] Cata JP, Chukka V, Wang H, Feng L, Gottumukkala V, Martinez F, Vaporciyan AA: Perioperative blood transfusions and survival in patients with non-small cell lung cancer: a retrospective study. *BMC anesthesiology* 2013, 13(1):42.

[38] Moir MS, Samy RN, Hanasono MM, Terris DJ: Autologous and heterologous blood transfusion in head and neck cancer surgery. *Archives of otolaryngology--head & neck surgery* 1999, 125(8):864-868.

[39] Busch OR, Hop WC, Hoynck van Papendrecht MA, Marquet RL, Jeekel J: Blood transfusions and prognosis in colorectal cancer. *The New England journal of medicine* 1993, 328(19):1372-1376.

[40] Fujimoto J, Okamoto E, Yamanaka N, Oriyama T, Furukawa K, Kawamura E, Tanaka T, Tomoda F: Efficacy of autotransfusion in

hepatectomy for hepatocellular carcinoma. *Archives of surgery* 1993, 128(9):1065-1069.

[41] Hirano T, Yamanaka J, Iimuro Y, Fujimoto J: Long-term safety of autotransfusion during hepatectomy for hepatocellular carcinoma. *Surgery today* 2005, 35(12):1042-1046.

[42] Liang TB, Li DL, Liang L, Li JJ, Bai XL, Yu W, Wang WL, Shen Y, Zhang M, Zheng SS: Intraoperative blood salvage during liver transplantation in patients with hepatocellular carcinoma: efficiency of leukocyte depletion filters in the removal of tumor cells. *Transplantation* 2008, 85(6):863-869.

[43] Bower MR, Ellis SF, Scoggins CR, McMasters KM, Martin RC: Phase II comparison study of intraoperative autotransfusion for major oncologic procedures. *Annals of surgical oncology* 2011, 18(1):166-173.

[44] Muscari F, Suc B, Vigouroux D, Duffas JP, Migueres I, Mathieu A, Lavayssiere L, Rostaing L, Fourtanier G: Blood salvage autotransfusion during transplantation for hepatocarcinoma: does it increase the risk of neoplastic recurrence? *Transplant international : official journal of the European Society for Organ Transplantation* 2005, 18(11):1236-1239.

[45] Mirhashemi R, Averette HE, Deepika K, Estape R, Angioli R, Martin J, Rodriguez M, Penalver MA: The impact of intraoperative autologous blood transfusion during type III radical hysterectomy for early-stage cervical cancer. *American journal of obstetrics and gynecology* 1999, 181(6):1310-1315; discussion 1315-1316.

[46] van Hilten JA, van de Watering LM, van Bockel JH, van de Velde CJ, Kievit J, Brand R, van den Hout WB, Geelkerken RH, Roumen RM, Wesselink RM *et al*: Effects of transfusion with red cells filtered to remove leucocytes: randomised controlled trial in patients undergoing major surgery. *Bmj* 2004, 328(7451):1281.

[47] Lange MM, van Hilten JA, van de Watering LM, Bijnen BA, Roumen RM, Putter H, Brand A, van de Velde CJ, cooperative clinical investigators of the Cancer R, Blood Transfusion s *et al*: Leucocyte depletion of perioperative blood transfusion does not affect long-term survival and recurrence in patients with gastrointestinal cancer. *The British journal of surgery* 2009, 96(7):734-740.

[48] Mynster T, Nielsen HJ, Danish RCCSG: Storage time of transfused blood and disease recurrence after colorectal cancer surgery. *Diseases of the colon and rectum* 2001, 44(7):955-964.

[49] Cata JP, Klein EA, Hoeltge GA, Dalton JE, Mascha E, O'Hara J, Russell A, Kurz A, Ben-Elihayhu S, Sessler DI: Blood storage duration and

biochemical recurrence of cancer after radical prostatectomy. *Mayo Clinic proceedings Mayo Clinic* 2011, 86(2):120-127.

[50] Frank SM, Resar LM, Rothschild JA, Dackiw EA, Savage WJ, Ness PM: A novel method of data analysis for utilization of red blood cell transfusion. *Transfusion* 2013, 53(12):3052-3059.

[51] Theusinger OM, Felix C, Spahn DR: Strategies to reduce the use of blood products: a European perspective. *Current opinion in anaesthesiology* 2012, 25(1):59-65.

[52] Musallam KM, Tamim HM, Richards T, Spahn DR, Rosendaal FR, Habbal A, Khreiss M, Dahdaleh FS, Khavandi K, Sfeir PM *et al*: Preoperative anaemia and postoperative outcomes in non-cardiac surgery: a retrospective cohort study. *Lancet* 2011, 378(9800):1396-1407.

[53] Spahn DR, Goodnough LT: Alternatives to blood transfusion. *Lancet* 2013, 381(9880):1855-1865.

[54] Shander A, Javidroozi M: Strategies to reduce the use of blood products: a US perspective. *Current opinion in anaesthesiology* 2012, 25(1):50-58.

[55] Goodnough LT, Monk TG, Andriole GL: Erythropoietin therapy. *The New England journal of medicine* 1997, 336(13):933-938.

In: General and Abdominal Surgery
Editor: Kassandra Sarah Slavomir

ISBN: 978-1-63117-440-7
© 2014 Nova Science Publishers, Inc.

Chapter 6

Gastroesophageal Reflux Disease: Pathophysiological and Therapeutic Considerations

Evgenios Evgeniou[1], Panagiotis A. Dimitriadis[2],
Petros V. Vlastarakos[3], Ashley Walden[2]
and Rishi Sharma[2]*

[1]General Surgery Department, Wexham Park Hospital, Slough, UK
[2]Ear, Nose and Throat Department,
Luton and Dunstable Hospital, Luton, UK
[3]Ear, Nose and Throat Department, Lister Hospital, Stevenage, UK

Abstract

Gastroesophageal reflux disease (GERD) is a common disease that accounts for the majority of oesophageal pathology. Patients with GERD typically complain of heartburn, regurgitation and/ or dysphagia. Extra-oesophageal symptoms are common and can delay diagnosis and treatment. Several factors may contribute to GERD: Dysfunction of the antireflux barrier, increased oesophageal sensitivity and abnormal oesophageal motility or gastric emptying all play a part in its pathogenesis.

* Corresponding author: Panagiotis A. Dimitriadis. Address: 6 Theobald Crescent, Harrow, HA3 5NB, e-mail address: panagiotis.dimitriadis.09@ ucl.ac.uk.

Conservative management is successful in 90% of cases and focuses on lifestyle changes and gastric acid suppression. Proton Pump Inhibitors and histamine- 2- receptor antagonists offer symptomatic relief but their long-term use has been criticized. Other medical treatments (prokinetics, tricyclic anti-depressants) can theoretically improve the symptoms, but the evidence for their use in daily practice, is insufficient.

In specific cases, surgical treatment is indicated. Antireflux surgery aims to restore the gastroesophageal barrier and is an effective way of providing long-term treatment. Nissen fundoplication is the procedure of choice, where the gastric fundus is mobilized and wrapped around the oesophagus (360^{0}). Different variants of the traditional method (Toupet fundoplication, Belsey Mark IV repair or anterior fundoplication) are recommended in certain cases. Other laparoscopic techniques include the use of magnetic field or electrical stimulation to re-enforce the lower oesophageal sphincter.

Surgical treatment carries the risk of untoward side effects. Besides the common complications of any surgical procedure, fundoplication may be complicated by dysphagia, inability to vomit, increased flactulence, herniation of the repair into the chest and recurrence or persistence of problems.

1. Background

Gastroesophageal reflux disease (GERD) is a common disease that accounts for the majority of oesophageal pathology [1]. It can be defined as excessive amounts of reflux associated with significant symptoms or complications. In the United Kingdom, National Institute for Clinical Excellence (NICE) refers to GERD as endoscopically determined oesophagitis or endoscopy-negative reflux disease [2]. Moreover, GERD is a well-recognised risk factor for adenocarcinoma of the oesophagus [3, 4]. Savary Miller and Los Angeles classifications are commonly used to describe severity of GERD (Table 1). In the US, gastroesophageal reflux (GER) prompted 8.9 million outpatient clinic visits in 2009 [5]. Its prevalence in the Western world is high (20-40%) and is thought to be related to modern dietary habits and increasing prevalence of obesity [6-8]. Patients with GERD typically complain of heartburn, regurgitation and/ or dysphagia that can significantly impact on the quality of life of those affected [9]. Several factors may contribute to GERD, however, true knowledge about its exact aetiology is limited because of lack of valid, population-based studies of sufficient statistical power [6]. Most commonly, GERD is caused by a dysfunctional lower esophageal sphincter (LES) complex [1]. Genetics have bee postulated to play a role in the aetiology of GERD: A study that compared reflux symptoms in monozygotic and dizygotic twins concluded that genetic factors may contribute by upto 31% to the aetiology of symptomatic GERD [10].

Table 1. Savary- Miller and Los Angeles classifications of GERD

Savary-Miller classification		Los Angeles classification	
Grade	Features	Grade	Features
I	Erosions to 1 mucosal fold	A	Erosions <5mm on single folds
II	>1 erosions on >1 fold	B	Erosions >5mm on single folds
III	Circumferential erosions	C	Erosions across >1 folds <75% of circumference
IV	Ulceration, shortening or stricture formation	D	Erosions across >75% of circumference
V	Barrett's epithelium formation		

2. Basic Anatomy of the Oesophagus

The adult oesophagus is an 18 to 26cm long muscular tube that connects the pharynx to the stomach. It extends from the upper sphincter to the lower sphincter and has 3 distinct regions: a) cervical, b) thoracic and c) abdominal (figure 1). Its lumen is normally collapsed but distends to allow the passage of food bolus during swallowing. The pharyngoesophageal junction lies posteriorly to the inferior border of the cricoid cartilage (C5-6 vertebral level). It then descends anteriorly and pierces the diaphragm through the diaphragmatic hiatus (T10 vertebral level). It ends at the orifice of the cardia of the stomach (T11 vertebral level). The upper and lower oesophageal sphincters, that are located at the upper and lower ends of the oesophagus respectively, are two high-pressure zones of tonically contracted smooth muscle that are responsible for preventing food regurgitation.

The esophagus contains four characteristic layers (Figure 2):

a) Mucosa, which is the innermost layer, lining the lumen of the organ.
b) Submucosa that lies underneath the mucosa and contains blood vessels, lymphatics and nerve endings.
c) Muscularis propria, which is made up of a circular inner layer and a longitudinal outer layer of smooth muscle cells, and

d) Serosa, which is the outermost layer, consists of the visceral peritoneum.

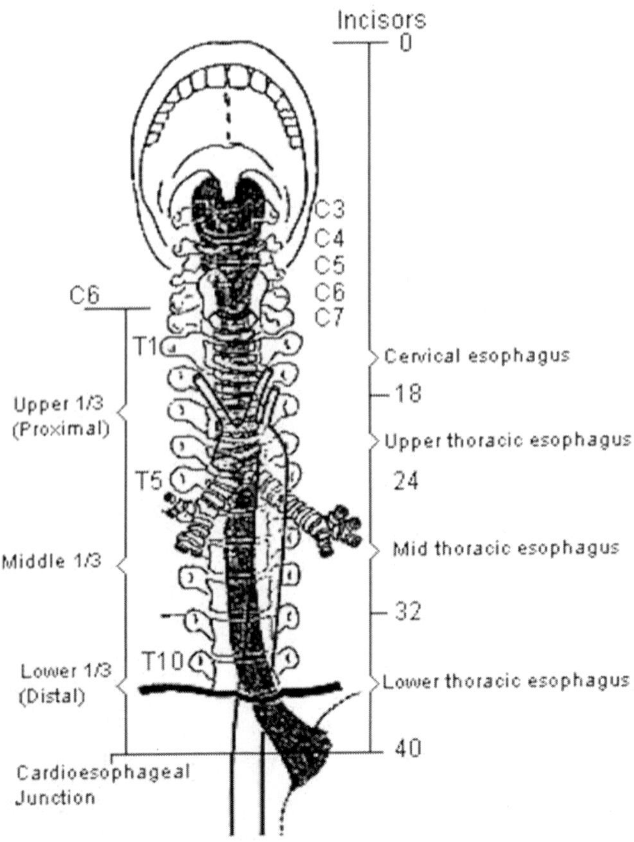

Figure 1. Position and relations of the oesophagus (source: Wikipedia[TM:] The free Encyclopedia).

With regards to esophagus' vasculature: The inferior thyroid artery supplies its cervical part; paired aortic oesophageal arteries supply the thoracic part and the left gastric artery along with a branch of the left phrenic artery supply the distal oesophagus. The proximal and distal parts of the oesophagus drain into the azygous system while its middle part drains into the left gastric vein, which is branch of the portal vein. There are extensive connections between the portal and systemic venous systems. With regards to its innervation, like the rest of the viscera, the oesophagus receives dual sensory innervation, namely parasympathetic and sympathetic; this regulates glandular secretion, vessel constriction and the activity of striated and smooth muscle. Vagal afferents (parasympathetic) transduce pressure into painful sensations but have no direct role in visceral pain transmission. The spinal afferents (sympathetic) are involved in mediating visceral nociception. The motor innervation of the oesophagus is predominantly via the vagal nerve.

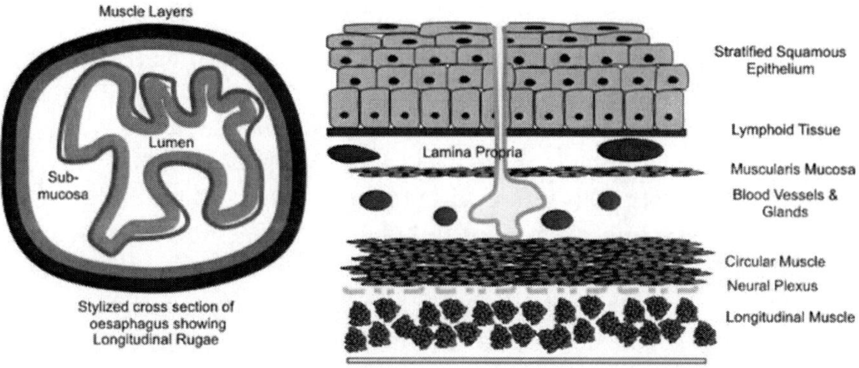

Figure 2. Layers of the oesophagus (source: Wikipedia$^{TM:}$ The free Encyclopedia).

3. Symptomatology and Pathophysiology

3.1. GERD's Symptomatology

Patients with GERD will commonly complain of heartburn, regurgitation and dysphagia. These symptoms are not exclusive to GERD so a detailed history and a thorough examination are essential to rule out any other pathology such as coronary artery disease, gallstone disease or cancer. The overall prevalence of these symptoms in overweight or obese subjects is high (37%) [11]. Heartburn is characterized by a retrosternal burning sensation that begins in the epigastrium and radiates upwards. It is known that dairy food, chocolate, coffee and alcohol as well as lying in the supine position can aggravate symptoms [12]. Regurgitation is the effortless backflow of gastric content into the pharynx or mouth. Symptoms worsen when lying supine or bending over and may be caused by an incompetent or obstructed gastroesophageal junction (GEJ). Night-time heartburn and sleep-related reflux play an important role in the development of oesophagitis and intestinal metaplasia (Barrett's oesophagus) [13]. Dysphagia is the medical term for the symptom of difficulty in swallowing. It affects 7-10% of patients over 50 years of age [14]. Although the term is non-specific, the investigating phycisian must rule out upper digestive tract pathology. Dysphagia is classified into 3 major types: a) oropharyngeal (difficulty transferring the food from mouth to oesophagus), b) oesophageal (sensation of food being stuck in lower chest) and c) functional (no organic cause for dysphagia can be found). However, GERD does not always present with the aforementioned typical symptoms: Chronic cough, dental erosion, asthma, recurrent pneumonia, chronic bronchitis, dysphonia, globus pharyngeus, otitis media and posterior laryngitis comprise common extraoesophageal manifestations of GERD, or "extraoesophageal syndrome" as is stated at the Montreal definition [15]. In a study of 47 patients with reflux-related cough, about 1/3 of them did not display any classic reflux symptoms (heartburn or indigestion) [16]. Similarly asthmatics display a greater prevalence of GERD than the general population but only about 2/3 of them present with typical reflux symptomatology [17]. In turn, symptoms commonly associated with asthma (e.g chest pain, cough) are commonly encountered in patients with GERD; so the nature of the association of the two clinical entities can be difficult to delineate. In a study of 10,689 patients presenting in an Emergency Department with acute chest pain, only 17% were found to have acute coronary syndrome whereas 55% had non-cardiac pathologies [18]. A good history taking may help distinguishing the non-cardiac chest pain from a true cardiac one. Chronic laryngitis is inflammation of the larynx that lasts more than 3 weeks. Cigarette smoke or other irritants trigger most cases of laryngitis. When the individual does not give a clear prodromal history, gastric reflux must be suspected. Laryngo-pharyngeal reflux (LPR) represents a controversial topic for both diagnosis and treatment. Several studies have shown that up to 10% of the patients presenting to ENT outpatient clinics may suffer from LPR [19 20]. The presenting complaint of these patients may vary from a dry cough to sensation of something in the throat (FOSIT), the need to constantly clear their throat, post-nasal drip, dysphonia etc. LPR tends to occur during the daytime in the upright position, and is not associated with obesity [21]. In addition, it commonly presents with normal oesophageal motility, and most patients do not have oesophagitis as in GERD [22].

3.2. GERD's Pathophysiology

The precise mechanisms accounting for the generation of symptoms secondary to oesophageal pathology remain unclear. Significant insight has been acquired by recent studies, however. The lower oesophageal sphincter (LES) along with the crural diaphragm, the angle of His (angle between the oesophagus and fundus), the Gubaroff flap valve and the phrenoesophageal membrane create an effective barrier preventing retrograde of gastric fluid into the oesophagus. These muscles remain in tonic opposition and occasionally, as in case of swallowing or when the gastric fundus is distended with gas, these muscles relax to enable flow of contents into the stomach or venting of gas (belch) [23].

Lower Esophageal Sphincter (figure 3): The resting tone of that zone is 5-25mmHg, relative to the intragastric pressure; that varies throughout the day (after meals, during exercise or sleep) and between individuals. Table 2 shows normal manometric values of the LES from a sample of 50 individuals. In this study, most common mechanism for reflux is Transient Lower Oesophageal Sphincter Relaxations (TLOSR), which are independent from the relaxations occurring during swallowing. Postprandial gastric distention is suggested to determine TLSOR; increased frequency and duration of which contribute to reflux disease [25 26].

The crural diaphragm surrounds the distal oesophagus and provides an extrinsic component to the gastroesophageal barrier, increasing the high-pressure zone of the LES. This mechanism has an important role in reducing the gastric reflux following sudden increases of intra-abdominal pressure. Its efficiency is minimized during TLOSRs or in the presence of a hiatus hernia, a condition where a portion of the stomach will protrude into the thorax through the diaphragm [27, 28].

Table 2. Normal manometric characteristics of LES (n=50)
(modified by Jobe et al., 2010 [34])

Parameter	Median value	2.5[th] percentile	97.5[th] percentile
Overall length (cm)	3.6	2.1	5.6
Abdominal length (cm)	2	0.9	4.7
Pressure (mmHg)	13	5.8	27.7

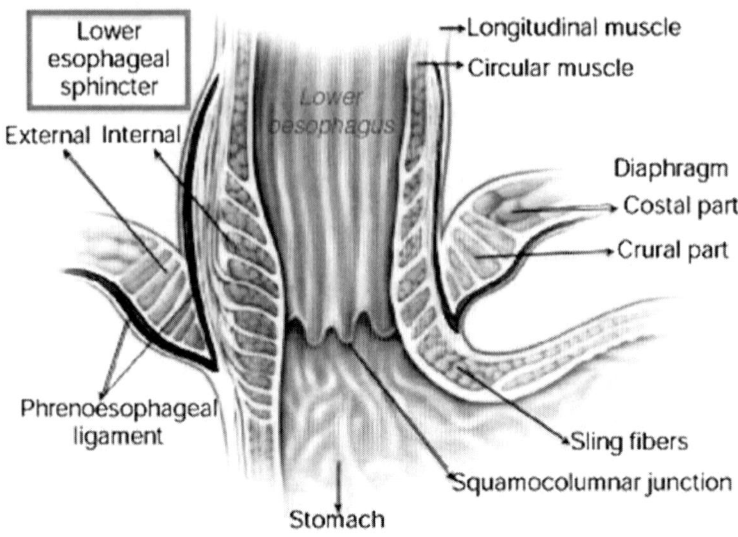

Figure 3. Lower oesophageal sphincter and its relations (modified from Mitall et al. [24]).

The Gubaroff valve (or plica cardiaca) normally sits at the GEJ and functions to maintain the angle of His and keep the distal part of the LES in the abdomen. Disruption of this flap valve and movement of the LES above the crural diaphragm result in significant relaxation of the high-pressure zone.

Normally pH in the stomach is reduced postprandially. Gastric and oesophageal pH monitoring showed that postprandial refluxate was more acidic than gastric contents. This would suggest that highly acidic unbuffered gastric juice is present at the GEJ (acid pocket) and is likely to contribute to the high prevalence of GERD at this site [29]. Some patients seem to be overly sensitive to the noxious stimuli of gastric reflux; they describe severe heartburn while their pH studies are within normal or slightly above the normal range. Enhanced visceral sensation may also play a part in the pathophysiology of GERD [30]. Factors that contribute to oesophageal hypersensitivity to acid are believed to be impaired mucosal barrier function, upregulation of peripheral nocicepstors and central sensitization [1].

The sequaelae of GERD may result from the direct harmful effects of gastric acid on the lining of the oesophagus, larynx or the airway tract. They include oesophagitis, oesophageal stricture formation, Barrett's oesophagus (see below), adenocarcinoma and progressive pulmonary fibrosis.

Recent studies show that severe oesophagitis and erosive oesophagitis are associated with pathological exposure to gastric acid combined with bile salts and pepsin [31] (Duodeno-Gastro-Oesophageal Reflux) as well as presence of a structurally defective sphincter. Erosive oesophagitis is found in almost half of patients with GERD and it is believed that worsening of mucosal injury is directly linked with subsequent deterioration of oesophageal motility [32, 33]. Going against this however is the fact that almost 40% of patients with a structurally defective sphincter have no obvious complications [34]. It seems that when the disease is confined to the LES, the oesophageal body can compensate with vigorous peristaltic contractions and prevent reflux. Eventually, loss of compensation occurs, which leads to reduced oesophageal clearance and increased risk of regurgitation, laryngeal involvement and aspiration [34].

Barrett's oesophagus is one of the most common premalignant lesions of the oesophagus in which normal squamous epithelium undergoes metaplasia and is replaced with a columnar type epithelium. Columnar epithelium is resistant to acid and is associated with improvement of symptoms of heartburn. A high prevalence of Barrett's oesophagus and oesophageal adenocarcinoma is seen in cases of increased pathological exposure of the oesophagus to the noxious bile acids and pancreatic enzymes. Complications of Barrett's oesophagus include oesophagitis, stricture, ulceration and dysplasia. The dysplasia can subsequently lead to neoplasia, a phenomenon strongly associated with chronic irritation of the mucosa from refluxed gastric and duodenal contents. Up to one third of patients found to have Barrett's oesophagus endoscopically, will have concomitant malignancy [34 35]. Oesophageal adenocarcinoma develops through progression of Barrett's oesophagus to low- and high-grade dysplasia and adenocarcinoma at a rate of 1% a year. Animal experiments have revealed a mutagenic potential of duodeno-gastric reflux to the oesophageal epithelium and linked it directly to oesophageal adenocarcinoma [36, 37].

3.3. Extraoesophageal Syndrome

Laryngeal symptoms (chronic cough, globus pharyngeus and dysphonia) are often secondary to gastric reflux. Oesophageal pH monitoring in patients with known GERD and laryngeal symptoms revealed significantly more proximal oesophageal acid exposure compared to patients with GERD but no laryngeal symptoms.

Reflux cough syndrome has a well established association with GERD is thought to be triggered by irritation of the upper respiratory tract by exposure to noxious agents present in the gastric and duodenal juice [38]. Moreover, chronic cough results to increased intra-abdominal pressure that in turn cycle through to increased reflux by overcoming the LES pressure [39]. Nonacidic reflux-associated cough has been suggested to play a role in cases where symptoms persist despite intensive medical treatment. In a large retrospective study that assessed the prevalence of GERD in patients presenting with chronic cough, pathologic oesophageal acid exposure was demonstrated in more than half of patients with chronic cough [40]. In a study of 183 patients with chronic cough, GERD was found to be the single cause of cough in 13% while in 56% of them GORD was a contributing factor [41].

Asthma and GERD are conditions commonly met in the general population and they often co-exist. However asthmatics have a much greater prevalence of GERD symptoms than would be expected by chance alone, with reported rates varying from 20-80% [42-44]. A significant proportion of asthmatics that have co-existant GERD (documented by pH studies) do not display classic GERD symptoms and are considered to have "silent GERD" [45]. There remains debate regarding the pathophysiology of this association. Suggested mechanisms by which GERD is speculated to worsen asthma include: a) aspiration of gastric contents that induces bronchoconstriction, vagal reflexes and chronic airway inflammation [46, 47] and b) vagally mediated reflex of bronchospasm due to chronic reflux and inflammation of the distal oesophagus [48]. The evidence supporting the former is based on clinical evidence that found a strong correlation between idiopathic pulmonary fibrosis and hiatal hernia [49]. The vagal reflex mechanism is supported by the bronchoconstriction that follows infusion of acid into the distal oesophagus. There is a shared embryologic origin of the vagus nerve and tracheo-oesophageal tract. This reflex is though to have developed to protect the aerodigestive system from the aspiration of gastric contents. In turn, asthma can worsen GERD symptoms: Bronchospasm and airway restriction can lead to hyperinflation and increased negative inspiratory pleural pressure that can both lead to a dysfunctional LES [50]. In LPR, laryngeal pathology results from small amounts of acid and pepsin causing damage to the sensitive laryngeal tissue, resulting in localised pathology.

The laryngeal epithelium protects itself against LPR to some extent by expressing a limited amount of carbonic anhydrase, which can catalyze the hydration of carbon dioxide (CO_2) to produce bicarbonate ($HCO3^-$). Moreover the proton pump associated with the parietal cells of the stomach is present in the seromucinous cells and ducts of the human larynx, with some variable expression [51]. Failure of these protective mechanisms leads cough and laryngospasm due to direct refluxate irritation as well as ciliary dysfunction and mucus accumulation that give the false sensation of post-nasal drip [52].

4. Treatment

4.1. Lifestyle Modifications

Conservative management is successful in 90% of cases and is centred on lifestyle changes and gastric acid suppression. A common approach in managing GERD is to encourage patients to change their lifestyle and alter their dietary habits. Increased risk of GERD is associated with consumption of high-fat meals, table salt and tobacco smoking [6]. Alcohol, coffee and tea consumption have previously been implicated in the genesis of GERD [53 54] however recent studies failed to confirm this association [6, 53]. On the other hand, a number of studies have shown that dietary fibers are associated with reduced risk of GERD [4 6]. Regular exercise of at least 30 minutes has been shown to be effective in reducing the risk of GERD possibly by strengthening the crural diaphragm and thus, improving the anti-reflux barrier [6]. GERD is highly prevalent in morbidly obese patients and a high Body Mass Index (BMI) is an independent risk factor for development of GERD [55]. Weight loss, especially in overweight or obese patients can lead to resolution of symptoms [11]. Elevating the head of the bed when sleeping is advised to patients whose symptoms are worse at night. Change of breathing pattern, from thoracic to abdominal, improved GERD as assessed by pH-measurement, Quality of Life (QoL) scores and PPI usage [56].

4.2.1. Medical Treatment of GERD

Despite the pathogenesis of GERD being secondary to anatomical disruption and abnormal motor function, the mainstay of treatment is suppression of the gastric acid production. In the United Kingdom, the National Institute for Clinical Excellence published guidelines on treatment of dyspepsia in adults in 2004 [2]. In its' guidance it suggested that surgical treatment should be pursued when medical treatment fails. Patients with GERD should be offered a trial of Proton Pump Inhibitors (PPIs) for one to two months. PPIs have been found to be more effective than Histamine Receptor Antagonists (H_2RAs) in managing GERD. In particular placebo was effective in 22%, H₂Ras in 39% and PPIs in 76% of patients [57, 58]. Patients with persistence of symptoms and severe oesophagitis may benefit from a double- dose PPI for one more month. Studies comparing different commonly used PPIs (omeprazole, esomeprazole, lansoprazole, pantoprazole and rabeprazole) concluded that esomeprazole at the standard dose provided more steady control of gastric acid at steady state [57, 58].

Most patients will have recurrence of symptoms following initial treatment. In these cases, a low-dose PPI should be offered with a limited number of repeat prescriptions. PPIs are associated with reduced risk of relapse of symptoms compared to H₂RAs (20% and 59% respectively). Antacid medications have a rapid onset of action and can be used on an "as required" basis where patients tailor their treatment to their needs. In cases where response to PPIs is inadequate, a trial of H₂RAs should be offered as individual subjects may respond better to these. Excessive use of antacids may cause constipation or diarrhea and in patients with chronic kidney injury, hypermagnesaemia or hyperaluminaemia [1]. Long-term use of antacids and chronic suppression of gastric acid secretion have been associated with atrophic gastritis, infection, *Clostridium difficile* diarrhea, increased risk of fractures, vitamin B12 and iron deficiencies [59-61].

4.2.2. Other Medical Treatment Options

Prokinetic agents enhance gastrointestinal motility by increasing the frequency of contractions in the small intestine or making them stronger, without disrupting their rhythm. Theoretically they could help relieve the symptoms of GERD by accelerating gastric emptying, or increasing the LES pressure. In a study of 20 individuals with GERD, metoclopramide and domperidone increased the LES pressure but had no effect on oesophageal body motility, duration of oesophageal exposure to acid and oesophageal clearance in comparison to placebo [62]. Cisapride is a prokinetic agent that increases motility of the upper gastrointestinal tract by acting directly as a serotonin-receptor agonist and indirectly as a parasympathomimetic. It was effective in managing GERD symptoms but is now withdrawn due to cardiac side effects [63].

Tricyclic anti-depressants have been found to decrease sensitivity to oesophageal distention in healthy individuals and provide pain relief in non-cardiac chest pain [64]. Citalopram (selective serotonin reuptake inhibitor) was found to increase the thresholds for perception and discomfort during balloon inflation test and oesophageal acid perfusion tests [65]. These agents may have a role in managing cases of oesophageal hypersensitivity but more studies are needed before their widespread use in treatment of GERD can be considered.

4.2.3. Medical Treatment of Extra-oesophageal Reflux Manifestations

Treatment of extra-oesophageal manifestations of GERD is essentially the same as for the oesophageal ones. It is likely to be more successful in the presence of oesophageal symptoms; a thorough consultation and reassurance of the patient is also imperative.

Eighty per cent of patients with GERD-related cough were successfully diagnosed and treated with a 4-6 week administration of a PPI alone or in combination with a prokinetic agent [41]. A follow-up of these patients shortly after initiation of PPI treatment is essential to avoid prolonged, often unnecessary use of such therapies. A positive response to an initial trial of PPIs seems to be the best indicator for eventual resolution [66]. Other studies have, however, failed to reveal any benefit to PPI therapy compared to placebo in individuals with chronic cough [67, 68].

4.3.1. Surgical Management of GERD

Surgery is considered complimentary to medical therapy in the management of GERD and tends to be reserved for patients with GERD refractory to medical treatment or for patients who are unwilling to be committed to a lifelong use of anti-reflux medication or are experiencing side effects form the treatment [1, 69, 70]. Surgery is infrequently undertaken for complications such as intestinal metaplasia, ulceration, or stenosis that develop or persist despite appropriate medical treatment [1].

Surgical anti-reflux options offer an alternative to life-long medications by addressing the cause of the disease.

The role of antireflux surgery is to correct the anatomical and physiological abnormalities that result in incompetence of the LES. In order to establish an effective LES pressure the GOJ is positioned and secured in the abdomen by creating a fundoplication above the sphincter [69]. A fundoplication also decreases the number of transient (not associated with a swallow) relaxations of the lower oesophageal sphincter, improves gastric emptying and creates a valve mechanism [71]. A systematic review by Catarci et al. in 2004 [72] has shown that laparoscopic fundoplication is as effective as open fundoplication in the management of GERD. Laparoscopic fundoplication is therefore considered the gold standard for the surgical management of GERD, combining the effective management of proven GERD with the benefits of laparoscopic surgery, such as reduced scaring and postoperative pain, reduced hospital stay and early return to normal activities [70]. Open fundoplication is offered when laparoscopy is contraindicated, such as in cases of uncontrollable coagulopathy and severe chronic obstructive pulmonary disease COPD). Previous upper abdominal operations, including previous open fundoplication, are considered a relative contraindications to a laparoscopic approach [69]. Although various types of anti-reflux surgical procedures have been described, the commonest are Nissen and Toupet fundoplications.

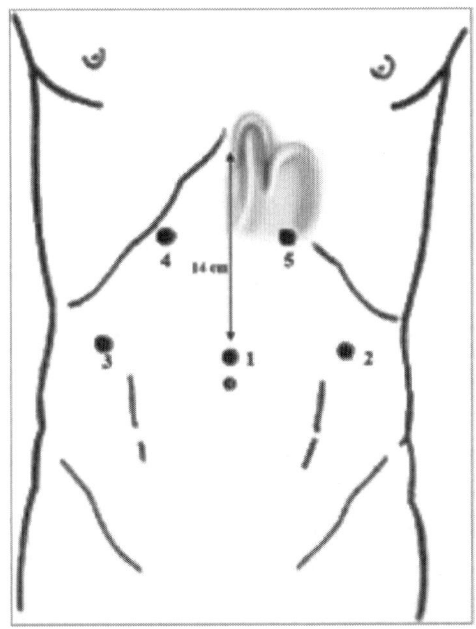

Figure 4. Placement of trocars during laparoscopic fundoplication (modified, by Allaix et. al. 2013 [73]).

Nissen fundoplication: Nissen is a total fundoplication. Five trocars are usually required for appropriate retraction and dissection, as shown in Figure 4 [73]. The gastrohepatic ligament and short gastric vessels are divided and the oesophagus is dissected from the right and left crus of the diaphragm, with care being taken to protect the anterior and posterior vagus nerve, which are usually retracted to the side using a penrose drain placed around them [69 73]. A 60 French Bougie is passed through the gastro-oesophageal junction and the fundus of the stomach is wrapped 360° around the oesophagus above the gastro-oesophageal junction by passing the left side of the fundus around the posterior aspect of the oesophagus and suturing it to the anterior aspect of the right side of the fundus and to the oesophagus (figure 5) The fundoplication is also then sutured to the inferior aspect of the diaphragm at the 11 and 2 o' clock positions. The completed fundoplication should be "floppy" in order to avoid postoperative dysphagia [74].

Toupet fundoplication: Toupet fundoplication is almost identical to Nissen fundoplication with the only difference being that the fundoplication is a 270° wrap rather than a 360° wrap. It is therefore a partial fundoplication [69].

Recent randomized controlled trials comparing the two types of fundoplication have concluded that although there is no statistically significant difference in the reduction of acid exposure between the two procedures, Toupet fundoplication is, however, associated with less dysphagia [75 76]. Toupet fundoplication is therefore the preferred option in patients with abnormal oesophageal peristalsis identified during preoperative oesophageal manometry [69].

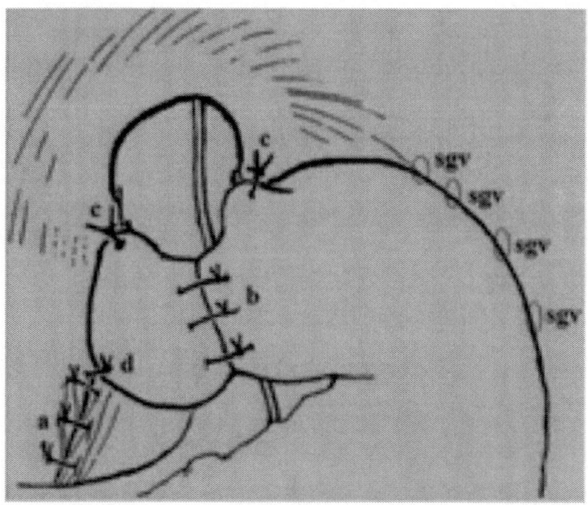

Figure 5. Total fundoplication; a closure of crura, b wrap, c coronal sutures, d posterior suture; sgv divided short gastric vessels (modified, by Allaix et al., 2013 [73]).

Fundoplication complications: The commonest complication is dysphagia due to a tight fundoplication or swelling at the gastro-oesophageal junction. Dysphagia has been reported to be present in 30-40% of the patients but it usually improves with time and only 5% of patients have dysphagia in the long term follow-up that will require dilatation or revision surgery [77]. Although most studies with short follow-up report a low rate of recurrence of anti-reflux symptoms following fundoplication [71 77], studies with long-term follow-up of patients have reported that 62% of patients who had undergone antireflux surgery continued to use medications for reflux symptom control 10 to 12 years following surgery [78]. If the use of anti-reflux medication following anti-reflux surgery is considered as a failure of the operation to control the symptoms, laparoscopic fundoplication is associated with a high failure rate in the long-term. However if the view is that surgery is an adjunct to medical management it can offer significant improvement in selected patients. Although laparoscopic fundoplication is considered a routine procedure, it does carry a mortality risk of 0.5-1% [79]. Other possible complications of fundoplication are shown on Table 3.

Table 3. Possible complications of fundoplication

Complications of surgical management of GERD	
Intraoperative	
Mortality	Pneumothorax
Bleeding	Subcutaneous emphysema
Perforation	
Postoperative	
Failure of treatment	Delayed gastric emptying
Dysphagia	Dumping
Postoperative nausea	Diarrhoea
Retching	Reflux Gastritis
Gas bloat	Wrap migration
Inability to belch	Paraesophageal herniation
Flatulence	

4.3.2. Endoscopic Management of Gastro-oesophageal Reflux Disease

Endoscopic treatments for gastro-oesophageal reflux disease offer the benefit of a non-pharmacologic treatment while avoiding a surgical skin incision and can be offered on an outpatient basis [69, 80].

Current, available techniques for endoscopic treatment of gastro-oesophageal reflux disease include suturing devices, injection of inert insoluble polymers and radiofrequency ablation [1,80]. All endoscopic techniques act by decreasing the compliance of the lower oesophageal sphincter. Additionally the endoscopic suturing techniques act by creating a valve mechanism and the radiofrequency methods act by reducing the incidence of transient lower esophageal sphincter relaxations through a neural mechanism. Although technically more demanding, endoscopic suturing techniques, such as Endocinch (Bard, Murray Hill, New Jersey) and Esophyx (Endogastric Solutions, Redmond, Washington) are the most popular endoscopic techniques. Possible complications of endoscopic suturing are chest pain, abdominal pain, pneumothorax, gastric perforation, gastric mucosal injury and pneumoperitoneum [80]. There is a lack of well-designed studies in the literature assessing the efficiency of endoscopic treatments in the management of gastro-oesophageal reflux disease, therefore the widespread use of these techniques cannot be currently recommended [1, 69, 79]. But these do represent an exciting possibility for less invasive procedural control of GERD in the future.

Conclusion

Gastroesophageal reflux disease (GERD) is a common disease that accounts for the majority of oesophageal pathology. Its prevalence in the Western world is high (20-40%) and is thought to be related to modern dietary habits and increasing prevalence of obesity. Patients with GERD will commonly complain of heartburn, regurgitation and dysphagia. Chronic cough, dental erosion, asthma, recurrent pneumonia, chronic bronchitis, dysphonia, globus pharyngeus, otitis media and posterior laryngitis comprise common extraoesophageal manifestations of GERD. The precise mechanisms accounting for the generation of symptoms secondary to oesophageal pathology remain unclear, however the Transient Lower Oesophageal Sphincter Relaxations seem to play an important role. Conservative management is successful in 90% of cases and is centred on lifestyle changes and gastric acid suppression. Surgery is considered complimentary to medical therapy in the management of GERD and tends to be reserved for patients with GERD refractory to medical treatment or for patients who are unwilling to be committed to a lifelong use of anti-reflux medication or are experiencing side effects form the treatment. Although various types of anti-reflux surgical procedures have been described, the commonest are Nissen and Toupet fundoplications. Although laparoscopic fundoplication is considered a routine procedure, it does carry a mortality risk of 0.5-1%.

References

[1] Bredenoord AJ, Pandolfino JE, Smout AJ. Gastro-oesophageal reflux disease. *Lancet* 2013;381(9881):1933-42.

[2] NICE. Dyspepsia: Management of dyspepsia in adults in primary care. *National Institute of Clinical Excellence, London* 2004.

[3] Lagergren J, Bergstrom R, Lindgren A, Nyren O. Symptomatic gastroesophageal reflux as a risk factor for esophageal adenocarcinoma. *N Engl J Med* 1999;340(11):825-31.

[4] De Ceglie A, Fisher DA, Filiberti R, Blanchi S, Conio M. Barrett's esophagus, esophageal and esophagogastric junction adenocarcinomas: the role of diet. *Clin Res Hepatol Gastroenterol* 2011;35(1):7-16.

[5] Peery AF, Dellon ES, Lund J, Crockett SD, McGowan CE, Bulsiewicz WJ, et al. Burden of gastrointestinal disease in the United States: 2012 update. *Gastroenterology* 2012;143(5):1179-87 e1-3.

[6] Nilsson M, Johnsen R, Ye W, Hveem K, Lagergren J. Lifestyle related risk factors in the aetiology of gastro-oesophageal reflux. *Gut* 2004;53(12):1730-5.

[7] Nilsson M, Lundegardh G, Carling L, Ye W, Lagergren J. Body mass and reflux oesophagitis: an oestrogen-dependent association? *Scand J Gastroenterol* 2002;37(6):626-30.

[8] Dent J, El-Serag HB, Wallander MA, Johansson S. Epidemiology of gastro-oesophageal reflux disease: a systematic review. *Gut* 2005;54(5):710-7.

[9] Isolauri J, Laippala P. Prevalence of symptoms suggestive of gastro-oesophageal reflux disease in an adult population. *Ann Med* 1995;27(1):67-70.

[10] Cameron AJ, Lagergren J, Henriksson C, Nyren O, Locke GR, 3rd, Pedersen NL. Gastroesophageal reflux disease in monozygotic and dizygotic twins. *Gastroenterology* 2002;122(1):55-9.

[11] Singh M, Lee J, Gupta N, Gaddam S, Smith BK, Wani SB, et al. Weight loss can lead to resolution of gastroesophageal reflux disease symptoms: a prospective intervention trial. *Obesity (Silver Spring)* 2013;21(2):284-90.

[12] Kaltenbach T, Crockett S, Gerson LB. Are lifestyle measures effective in patients with gastroesophageal reflux disease? An evidence-based approach. *Arch Intern Med* 2006;166(9):965-71.

[64] Peghini PL, Katz PO, Castell DO. Imipramine decreases oesophageal pain perception in human male volunteers. *Gut* 1998;42(6):807-13.

[65] Broekaert D, Fischler B, Sifrim D, Janssens J, Tack J. Influence of citalopram, a selective serotonin reuptake inhibitor, on oesophageal hypersensitivity: a double-blind, placebo-controlled study. *Aliment Pharmacol Ther* 2006;23(3):365-70.

[66] Baldi F, Cappiello R, Cavoli C, Ghersi S, Torresan F, Roda E. Proton pump inhibitor treatment of patients with gastroesophageal reflux-related chronic cough: a comparison between two different daily doses of lansoprazole. *World J Gastroenterol* 2006;12(1):82-8.

[67] Faruqi S, Molyneux ID, Fathi H, Wright C, Thompson R, Morice AH. Chronic cough and esomeprazole: a double-blind placebo-controlled parallel study. *Respirology* 2011;16(7):1150-6.

[68] Shaheen NJ, Crockett SD, Bright SD, Madanick RD, Buckmire R, Couch M, et al. Randomised clinical trial: high-dose acid suppression for chronic cough - a double-blind, placebo-controlled study. *Aliment Pharmacol Ther* 2011;33(2):225-34.

[69] Smith CD. Antireflux surgery. *Surg Clin North Am* 2008;88(5): 943-58, v.

[70] Lundell L. Surgical therapy of gastro-oesophageal reflux disease. *Best Pract Res Clin Gastroenterol* 2010;24(6):947-59.

[71] Horgan S, Pellegrini CA. Surgical treatment of gastroesophageal reflux disease. *Surg Clin North Am* 1997;77(5):1063-82.

[72] Catarci M, Gentileschi P, Papi C, Carrara A, Marrese R, Gaspari AL, et al. Evidence-based appraisal of antireflux fundoplication. *Ann Surg* 2004;239(3):325-37.

[73] Allaix ME, Herbella FA, Patti MG. Laparoscopic total fundoplication for gastroesophageal reflux disease. How I do it. *J Gastrointest Surg* 2013;17(4):822-8.

[74] Richardson WS, Trus TL, Hunter JG. Laparoscopic antireflux surgery. *Surg Clin North Am* 1996;76(3):437-50.

[75] Broeders JA, Roks DJ, Ahmed Ali U, Watson DI, Baigrie RJ, Cao Z, et al. Laparoscopic anterior 180-degree versus nissen fundoplication for gastroesophageal reflux disease: systematic review and meta-analysis of randomized clinical trials. *Ann Surg* 2013;257(5):850-9.

[76] Tan G, Yang Z, Wang Z. Meta-analysis of laparoscopic total (Nissen) versus posterior (Toupet) fundoplication for gastro-oesophageal reflux disease based on randomized clinical trials. *ANZ J Surg* 2011;81(4):246-52.

[77] Hinder RA, Klingler PJ, Perdikis G, Smith SL. Management of the failed antireflux operation. *Surg Clin North Am* 1997;77(5):1083-98.

[78] Spechler SJ, Lee E, Ahnen D, Goyal RK, Hirano I, Ramirez F, et al. Long-term outcome of medical and surgical therapies for gastroesophageal reflux disease: follow-up of a randomized controlled trial. *JAMA* 2001;285(18):2331-8.

[79] Moayyedi P, Talley NJ. Gastro-oesophageal reflux disease. *Lancet* 2006;367(9528):2086-100.

[80] de Hoyos A, Fernando HC. Endoscopic therapies for gastroesophageal reflux disease. *Surg Clin North Am* 2005;85(3):465-81, viii.

In: General and Abdominal Surgery
Editor: Kassandra Sarah Slavomir

ISBN: 978-1-63117-440-7
© 2014 Nova Science Publishers, Inc.

Chapter 7

Hydatid Liver Cyst

Jitendra Kumar Kushwaha, Abhinav Arun Sonkar,
Kulranjan Singh, Akshay Anand
and Rajni Gupta*
King George's Medical University, Lucknow, India

Abstract

Echinococcosis (hydatid disease) a Zoonosis caused by larval stage of Echinococcus granulosus (also known as Taenia echinococcus). Humans are accidental intermediate hosts,whwreas animals can be both intermediate and definitive hosts. The two main types of hydatid disease are caused by E. granulosus and E. multilocularis. E. granulosus is the most common type of hydatid disease in humans and commonly seen in the Mediterranean, South America, South Africa, Middle east and Australia. Whereas E.multilocularis producing alveolar hydatid disease (alveolar echinococcosis -AE) is limited to certain area of northern hemisphere.

In humans 50-75% of cyst occur in Liver,25% are located in lungs and less frequently to spleen, kidney, bones, and the brain. Although primary extra-hepatic locations are less common (or even rare in AE), any other organ may be involved. Secondary echinococcosis can develop in the same or other organs. Although less common, AE poses a far more serious problem due to the infiltrative nature of its cysts and its greater

---

* Corresponding Author.

ability to metastasise; it has to be regarded as a malignant disease carrying a mortality of up to 90% in untreated cases. Unless otherwise stated in text we refer to E. granulosus.

The modern treatment of hydatid cyst of the liver varies from surgical intervention to percutaneous drainage or medical therapy. Surgery is still the treatment of choice and can be performed by the conventional or laparoscopic approach. However, laparoscopic approach leads to an important rate of recurrence of the disease. Percutaneous Aspiration-Injection-Reaspiration Drainage (PAIR) seems to be a better alternative to surgery in selected cases.

1. Introduction

Hydatid disease, or echinococcosis, is a widespread zoonotic parasitic disease caused by a tapeworm that continues to be a clinical and public health problem worldwide.. Hydatid disease is most frequently caused by *Echinococcus granulosus*, and the liver is the most commonly involved organ in more than half of patients, although it may affect any part of the body, occurring either as a primary or secondary event. [1] The life cycle of *Echinococcus* requires a dog as a definitive host, and an intermediate host, which is commonly sheep. Humans become accidental intermediate hosts when they become infected after ingesting ova passed in dog feces.

Surgery is the treatment of choice for complicated cases, but uncomplicated cysts located in easily accessible areas of liver have been treated successfully by laparoscopy. Medical treatment alone is effective in selected patients. Percutaneous treatment techniques represent an important therapeutic advance in the treatment of hydatid disease. Several complications may occur during the course of the disease, the most frequent and severe of which are secondary infection of the cyst cavity, biliary fistula causing jaundice and cholangitis, and rupture of the cyst into the peritoneal or pleural cavity.

2. Etiology

Earlier epidemiologic studies have led to the recognition of only four clinically important species: *E. granulosus, E. multilocularis (E. alveolaris), E. oligarthrus,* and *E. vogeli* [2] with the discovery of a new strain, *E. shiquicus,* identified on the Tibetan plateau. [1] *E. granulosus* is the most common with *E. multilocularis* is responsible for a rare and aggressive form of hydatid disease.

E. granulosus, a hermaphroditic tapeworm consists of a head, or *scolex,* and a body, or *strobila,* with three or four proglottids. The eggs contain a hexacanth embryo that has three pairs of hooklets. The life cycle (Figure 1) of *E. granulosus* requires two hosts, a carnivore and an herbivore. Dog is the most common definitive host for *E. granulosus*. Worms release large numbers of infected eggs that pass out in the dog feces and contaminate soil, water, and plants. The eggs are ingested by the intermediate host (humans are accidental intermediate hosts), the eggs hatch, and the embryo migrates through the intestinal wall into the portal system. Most embryos lodge in the liver, mainly in the right lobe because of preferential portal flow where they evolve into hydatid cysts within months to years. Embryos may escape this first filter and lodge in the capillaries of the lung. Rarely a small percentage of embryos find their way into the systemic circulation and involve other organs, including the spleen, kidney, brain, bone, or any other site. In the liver, the parasite develops into the larval stage, the hydatid cyst, which is filled with fluid and contains hundreds of protoscolices. [3]

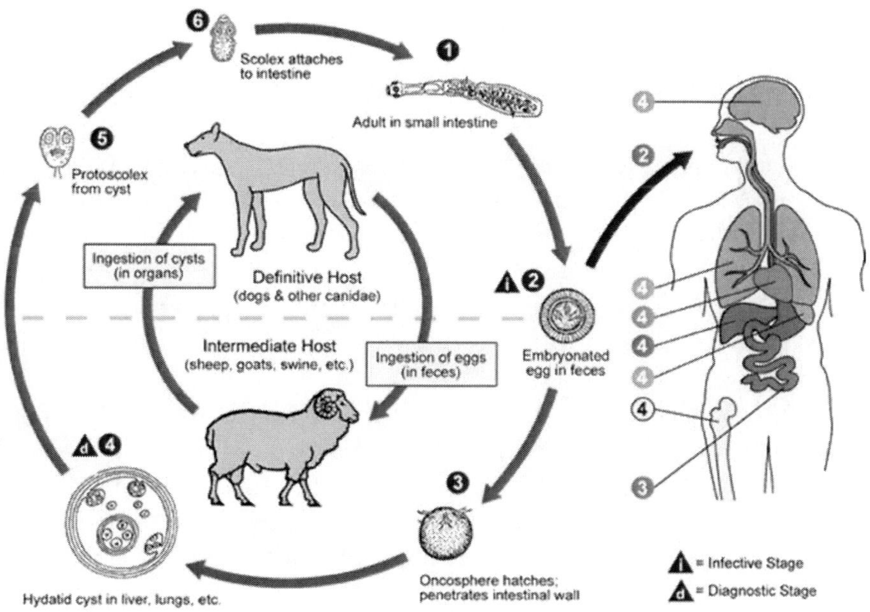

Figure 1. Life cycle of Echinococcus.

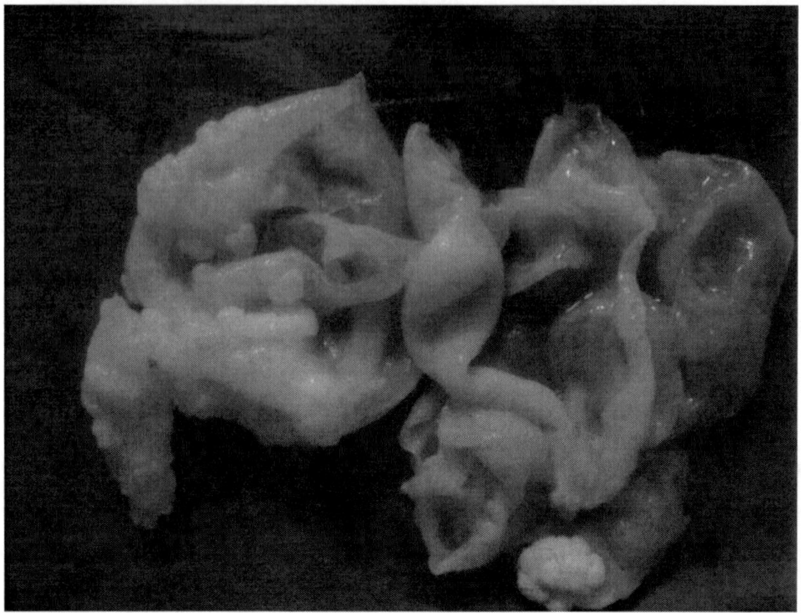

Figure 2. Hepatic hydatid cyst.

3. Cyst

When the parasite reaches the liver parenchyma, it develops into a cystic larval phase (Figure 2). The mature *E. granulosus* cyst consists of three layers: a *germinal layer,* a *laminated layer,* and an *ectocyst.* The inner, germinal layer surrounds the fluid-filled central hydatid cavity and in turn is surrounded by the laminated layer. These two layers together form the *endocyst.* Compression of the host tissue around the endocyst produces a fibrous layer known as the *ectocyst* or *pericyst.*

The germinal layer is the living component of the parasite. Undifferentiated cells in the germinal layer produce invaginations into the cyst cavity, forming brood capsules that contain protoscolices, which are released into the cyst fluid. The germinal membrane secretes fluid into the cyst and is the source of daughter cysts (endogenous vesiculation). Daughter cysts have a structure similar to the mother cysts.

The ectocyst or pericyst is a fibrous capsule that develops from host tissue response as an inflammatory reaction to the tapeworm. Rupture of hydatid fluid produces implantation of protoscolices and secondary cysts on surrounding viscera, known as *secondary hydatidosis.* [3] Although any segment of the liver can be involved, the location of liver hydatid cysts seems to be related to the respective volume of each lobe of the liver; thus a higher involvement of the right lobe is observed, especially in segments VII and VIII. [6]

4. Complications

Hydatid cysts in the liver may cause symptoms as a result of direct pressure, from the inflammatory reaction around the cyst, from distortion of neighboring structures or viscera, or as a result of erosion into the bile duct, pleural space, or peritoneal cavity. Rarely the cyst may rupture into the bronchial tree, pericardium, or digestive tract. Depending on the location, large cysts can cause compression of the adjacent bile ducts, portal or hepatic veins, or vena cava that causes obstructive jaundice, portal hypertension, or Budd-Chiari syndrome respectively. [7]

Cysts may become infected and clinical presentation is similar to a pyogenic liver abscess.

Intrabiliary rupture is the most common complication of liver hydatid cysts [8, 9] with minor or major cystobiliary communications.. The reported incidence of clinically evident cystobiliary communications rates varies from 2.6% to 28.6%. [10, 11]. Atli and colleagues [12] have found that a cyst diameter greater than 10 cm was an independent clinical predictor for the presence of intrabiliary rupture. Endoscopic retrograde cholangiopancreatography (ERCP) is useful to confirm biliary obstruction that results from hydatid material and facilitate treatment with an endoscopic sphincterotomy and extraction of the hydatid debris with a balloon or basket. [13] Intraperitoneal rupture of a hydatid cyst though spontaneous is an uncommon clinical presentation, even in endemic regions, with an incidence ranging from 1% to 8%. [14]

Rupture into the gastrointestinal tract that involves the stomach and the duodenum has been reported. [15] Isolated cases of rupture of liver hydatid cysts into the pericardium [16] and into large vessels, including the inferior vena cava, have also been described. [17]

5. Diagnosis

The diagnosis of hydatid cyst is based on a detailed history, quality imaging, and serology.

5.1. Clinical Symptoms

Cysts less than 5cm and uncomplicated cysts usually are asymptomatic and detected incidentally during a radiologic examination of the upper abdomen or right upper quadrant. Larger cyst may cause moderate pain in the right upper quadrant or in the right lower chest. Acute abdominal pain usually indicates an infected hydatid cyst or rupture into the peritoneal cavity. When antigenic cyst fluid is released into the circulation, especially after rupture into the peritoneal cavity, a variety of acute allergic manifestations may occur, such as urticaria, anaphylactic attacks, or episodes of asthma and sudden death. [18] Clinical features of rupture into the biliary tree are recurrent colicky pain and jaundice, with features resembling cholangitis.

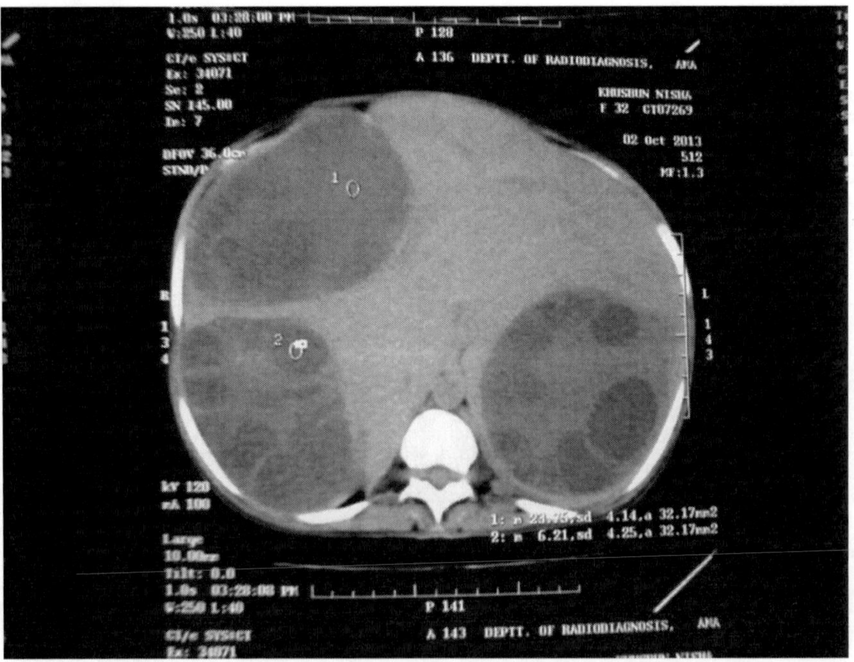

Figure 3. CT Scan showing hepatic hydatid cyst.

5.2. Laboratory Tests

Cholestatic enzymes, such as alkaline phosphatase and GGT, can be mildly elevated in about one third of patients, especially in patients with biliary compression [19] with elevated bilirubin levels (>1 mg/dL) with elevated alkaline phosphatase and GGT levels, highly suggesting a cystobiliary communication. White blood cell counts are elevated only if the cyst has become secondarily infected. Eosinophilia (>3%) occurs in 25% to 45% of patients. Serum immunoglobulin levels are elevated in only 31% of affected patients. [19]

5.3. Radiology

Ultrasound and Computed Tomography

USG is the preferred first-line imaging method for hydatid liver cyst assessment followed by CT (Figure 3), which gives more precise information regarding the detailed morphology of the cyst, including size, location, number, and relationship to adjacent structures. [20]

Hydatid cysts appear as well-defined, circumscribed cystic lesions with a clear membrane. [20, 21]

MRI

In cysts with biliary complications, MR cholangiography can provide good visualization of the intrahepatic and extrahepatic biliary tree and its relationship with the hydatid cyst and cystobiliary communications thus MRI is more specific in comparison to CT, especially if intracystic fat density is present, which suggests cystobiliary communication. [22, 23]

5.4. Serology

Immunoelectrophoresis: The diagnostic value of hydatidosis with immunoelectrophoresis ranges from 91% to 94% for hepatic cysts and 69% to 70% for pulmonary cysts. [24]

Enzyme-Linked Immunosorbent Assay: Sensitivities for enzyme-linked immunosorbent assay (ELISA) vary from 64% to 100% depending on the antigens used. [23]

Blotting: Western blotting with purified antigens has proved to be very useful in the diagnosis and postsurgical monitoring of hydatidosis patients. Purified fractions enriched in antigens 5 and B and in glycoprotein yield a sensitivity of 95% and specificity of 100%. [25, 26]

6. Principles of Management

In general, hydatid disease is a public health problem, especially in developing countries, and the specific treatment selected may depend on social circumstances and the medical expertise available. [17] Three treatment options are currently available for hydatid disease of the liver: surgery, which remains the most efficient treatment and the therapy of choice; percutaneous aspiration(PAIR); and medical treatment.

6.1. Surgical Treatment

The surgical management of hydatid liver disease includes a variety of different techniques, ranging from simple evacuation to major liver resection. [27] These techniques can be divided into two broad groups, *conservative (involving* inactivation of protoscolices and removal of the cyst contents) and *radical (demanding* total excision of the cyst and pericyst layers along with a portion of surrounding liver). [28]

6.1.1. Conservative Surgery: Principles and Techniques

Cystectomy is the safest and simplest surgical approach [28]. A full laparotomy is performed, paying particular attention to potential sites of dissemination, including the omentum and pelvis. [28] The characterisitic shiny white adventitial surface of a hydatid cyst is usually easily identified..

The area around the cyst is carefully isolated by gauze packs: the first layer is soaked with normal saline, and the second layer is soaked with a scolicidal solution. The cyst wall is pierced with a large-gauge needle and aspirated. If the cyst fluid is completely clear and not bile stained, turbid, or infected, scolicidal solution(10-15% normal saline) can be safely injected and left in the cavity for several minutes and then is reaspirated; this process is repeated twice. [29] The cyst is decompressed again by aspiration. Once the liquid has been drained, the laminated membrane collapses into the cavity, and the cyst contents can be evacuated. When all visible daughter cysts have been evacuated, the cavity is lavaged with warm saline, and the redundant portion of the cyst roof is excised and the cut edges are oversewn with a running mattress suture with an absorbable suture material.

widely used scolicidal agents include hypertonic saline, fresh half-strength Eusol, 0.5% silver nitrate, and hydrogen peroxide. Hypertonic saline has been widely used in the past because of its availability and effective scolicidal properties. [30]

Absolute alcohol has been used by interventional radiologists for the percutaneous treatment of hydatid cysts to produce sclerosis of the cyst cavity [31], but it is not effective on protoscolices inside daughter cysts [30]. Formalin is no longer used because of a high propensity to induce caustic sclerosing cholangitis. Any obvious biliary orifices should be sutured to prevent postoperative biliary leakage, fistula, and cavity infections. The omentum is mobilized from the transverse colon with sufficient mobility to pack the cavity and obliterate the dead space, and it is sutured to tether the omentum in place. [32, 33]

6.1.2. Pericystectomy

Also called *radical cystectomy, capsulectomy, total pericystectomy,* and *cystopericystectomy,* it involves complete removal of the hydatid cyst. By creating a surgical plane just outside the pericyst layer without opening the cyst, the parasite and the adventitial layer are excised en bloc [28, 33]

6.1.3. Radical Surgery: Liver Resection

The indications for hepatic resection for liver hydatid cysts are rare. Hepatic resection is the only surgical therapy for *E. multilocularis,* but it is inappropriately radical for *E. granulosus.* Other sparse indications for liver resection are when the remaining parenchyma of a liver lobe is atrophic as a result of biliary obstruction, or when a large bile leak that cannot be safely managed with a surgical drainage procedure is present [9, 28]

6.1.4. Role of Laparoscopy

Although the laparoscopic approach to this disease offers some advantages, laparoscopic hydatid surgery has not gained a wide acceptance due to a large learning curve. Technical limitations of the laparoscopic approach are the limited area for manipulation, intricacy in controlling spillage during puncture, and difficulty in aspirating the thick, degenerated cyst contents.

6.2. Percutaneous Treatment(PAIR)

Recently USG or CT Guided **P**ercutaneous **A**spiration, **I**nstillation of scolicidal agent and **R**easpiration treatment of hydatid cysts has been encouraged to aspirate and treat hydatid cysts of the liver using. [11]

Patients are given albendazole before and after the procedure for prophylaxis. Under local anesthesia, a fine needle is inserted into the cystic cavity through normal liver tissue with US or CT guidance. As much fluid as possible is aspirated and, on completion, a protoscolicidal agent is injected into the cavity. After 15 minutes, as much fluid as possible is reaspirated and the needle is withdrawn.

6.3. Chemotherapy

Mebendazole was introduced first, but albendazole became the drug of choice because of its superior absorption in the gastrointestinal tract and better clinical results. [34]

It has been shown that a success rate of 74% can be expected in patients with single cysts treated for 3 to 6 months. Treatment is usually administered in three or four courses lasting 4 weeks separated by a 2-week interval. Three courses are routinely recommended, in agreement with viability data suggesting that a maximum benefit is not reached with less than 3 months of therapy [36, 35].

References

[1]   Shaw, Bornman, Krige, 2006. Shaw JM, Bornman PC, Krige JEJ: Hydatid disease of the liver. *S. Afr. J. Surg.* 2006; 44:70-77.

[2]   Thompson 2001. Thompson RCA: *Echinococcosis.* In: Gillespie S, Pearson RD, ed. *Principles and Practice of Clinical Parasitology,* Chichester, England: John Wiley & Sons; 2001:587-612.

[3]   Krige, Beckingham, 2001. Krige JEJ, Beckingham IJ: *Liver abscesses and hydatid disease* In: Beckingham IJ, ed. *ABC of Liver, Pancreas, and Gallbladder,* London: British Medical Journal Publishing Group; 2001:29-32.

[4]   Richards, 1992. Richards KS: *Biology of Echinococcus and diagnosis of hydatid disease.* In: Morris DL, Richards KS, ed. *Hydatid Disease:*

Current Medical and Surgical Management, Oxford: UK, Butterworth Heinemann; 1992:1-24.

[5] Watson-Jones, Macpherson, 1988. Watson-Jones DL, Macpherson CN: Hydatid disease in the Turkana district of Kenya. VI. Man–dog contact and its role in the transmission and control of hydatidosis amongst the Turkana. *Ann. Trop. Med. Parasitol.* 1988; 82:343-356.

[6] Kayaalp et al., 2003. Kayaalp C, et al: Distribution of hydatid cysts into the liver with reference to cystobiliary communications and cavity-related complications. *Am. J. Surg.* 2003; 185:175-179.

[7] Moreno-Gonzalez et al., 1994. Moreno-Gonzalez E, et al: Liver transplantation for Echinococcus granulosus hydatid disease. *Transplantation* 1994; 58:797-800.

[8] Iscan, Duren, 1991. Iscan M, Duren M: Endoscopic sphincterotomy in the management of postoperative complications of hepatic hydatid disease. *Endoscopy* 1991; 23:282-283.

[9] Yilmaz, Gokok, 1990. Yilmaz E, Gokok N: Hydatid disease of the liver: current surgical management. *Br J Clin* 1990; 44:612-615.

[10] Langer et al., 1984. Langer JC, et al: Diagnosis and management of hydatid disease of the liver: a 15-year North American experience. *Ann. Surg.* 1984; 199:412-417.

[11] Akhan, Ozmen, 1999. Akhan O, Ozmen MN: Percutaneous treatment of liver hydatid cysts. *Eur. J. Radiol.* 1999; 32:76-85.

[12] Atli et al., 2001. Atli M, et al: Intrabiliary rupture of a hepatic hydatid cyst: associated clinical factors and proper management. *Arch. Surg.* 2001; 136:1249-1255.

[13] Ozaslan, Bayraktar, 2002. Ozaslan E, Bayraktar Y: Endoscopic therapy in the management of hepatobiliary hydatid disease. *J. Clin. Gastroenterol.* 2002; 35:160-174.

[14] Sozuer et al., 2002. Sozuer EM, et al: The perforation problem in hydatid disease. *Am. J. Trop. Med. Hyg.* 2002; 66:575-577.

[15] Diez Valladares et al., 1998. Diez Valladares L, et al: Hydatid liver cyst perforation into the digestive tract. *Hepatogastroenterology* 1998; 45:2110-2114.

[16] Thameur et al., 2001. Thameur H, et al: Cardiopericardial hydatid cysts. *World J. Surg.* 2001; 25:58-67.

[17] Karunajeewa et al., 2002. Karunajeewa HA, et al: Hydatid disease invading the inferior vena cava: successful combined medical and surgical treatment. *Aust. N. Z. J. Surg.* 2002; 72:159-160.

[18] Vuitton, 2004. Vuitton DA: Echinococcosis and allergy. *Clin. Rev. Allergy Immunol.* 2004; 26:93-104.

[19] Kayaalp et al., 2002. Kayaalp C, et al: Biliary complications after hydatid liver surgery: incidence and risk factors. *J. Gastrointest. Surg.* 2002; 6:706-712.

[20] Beggs, 1983. Beggs I: The radiological appearances of hydatid disease of the liver. *Clin. Radiol.* 1983; 34:555-563.

[21] Gharbi et al., 1981. Gharbi HA, et al: Ultrasound examination of the hydatic liver. *Radiology* 1981; 139:459-463.

[22] Pedrosa et al., 2000. Pedrosa I, et al: Hydatid disease: radiologic and pathologic features and complications. *Radiographics* 2000; 20:795-817.

[23] Basaran et al., 2005. Basaran C, et al: Fat-containing lesions of the liver: cross-sectional imaging findings with emphasis on MRI. *AJR Am. J. Roentgenol.* 2005; 184:1103-1110.

[24] Varela-Diaz et al., 1983. Varela-Diaz VM, et al: Immunodiagnosis of human hydatid disease: applications and contributions to a control program in Argentina. *Am. J. Trop. Med. Hyg.* 1983; 32:1079-1087.

[25] Zhang et al., 2003. Zhang W, et al: Concepts in immunology and diagnosis of hydatid disease. *Clin. Microbiol. Rev.* 2003; 16:18-36.

[26] Sbihi et al., 1996. Sbihi Y, et al: Serologic recognition of hydatid cyst antigens using different purification methods. *Diagn. Microbiol. Infect. Dis.* 1996; 24:205-211.

[27] Buttenschoen, Buttenschoen, 2003. Buttenschoen K, Buttenschoen D: Echinococcus granulosus infection: the challenge of surgical treatment. *Langenbecks Arch. Surg.* 2003; 388:218-230.

[28] Morris, 1992. Morris DL: *Surgical management of hepatic hydatid cyst.* In: Morris DL, Richards KS, ed. *Hydatid Disease: Current Medical and Surgical Management*, Oxford: Butterworth Heinemann; 1992:57-75.

[29] Terblanche, Krige, 1998. Terblanche J, Krige JEJ: *The management of hepatic Echinococcus.* In: Cameron JL, ed. *Current Surgical Therapy*, 6th ed. Baltimore: Mosby; 1998:326-330.

[30] Kayaalp et al., 1999. Kayaalp C, et al: Türkiye'de kist hidatik cerrahisinde skolisidal ve perioperatif benzimidazol kullanimi. *Ankara Cerrahi Dergisi* 1999; 4:201-207.

[31] Akhan O, et al: Percutaneous treatment of abdominal hydatid cysts with hypertonic saline and alcohol: an experimental study in sheep. *Invest. Radiol.* 1993; 28:121-127.

[32] Abu Zeid et al., 1998. Abu Zeid M, et al: Surgical treatment of hepatic hydatid cysts. *Hepatogastroenterology* 1998; 45:1802-1806.

Index

<table>
<tr><td>

A

Abraham, 29
access, 33
accounting, 125, 135
acid, ix, 7, 9, 13, 14, 21, 22, 25, 39, 41, 57,
 120, 126, 127, 128, 129, 130, 133, 135,
 138, 139, 140, 141
acid perfusion test, 130
acidic, 82, 126, 138
acidity, 140
ACTH, 81
action potential, 67
acute lung injury, ix, 101, 105, 114
adaptation, 79
adaptive immunity, ix, 101
adenocarcinoma, 88, 96, 97, 108, 113, 115,
 120, 126, 127, 136
adenoma, 87
adhesion, 40, 87
adipocyte, vii, 2, 3, 4, 5, 7, 8, 12, 13, 14, 16,
 17, 23, 27
adiponectin, 3, 4, 5, 8, 17, 19
adipose, vii, 1, 2, 3, 4, 5, 6, 7, 8, 9, 10, 12,
 14, 15, 16, 17, 18, 19, 21, 22, 23, 24, 25,
 27, 28, 29
adipose tissue, vii, 1, 2, 3, 4, 5, 6, 7, 8, 9,
 10, 12, 14, 15, 16, 17, 18, 19, 21, 22, 23,
 24, 25, 27, 28, 29
adiposity, 4, 7, 15, 19

</td><td>

adrenaline, 94
adults, 24, 46, 72, 129, 136, 140
adverse event, 114
aetiology, 120, 136
afferent nerve, 80
Africa, 54
African-American, 59
age, viii, 9, 25, 36, 37, 53, 55, 56, 57, 59,
 61, 68, 72, 106, 124
aging population, 54
agonist, 130
airway inflammation, 128
albumin, 82
alertness, 80
allergic reaction, 103, 111
allergy, 19, 154
American Heart Association, 62
American Red Cross, 102
amino, 80, 82
amino acid, 80, 82
ampulla, 109
analgesic, 84, 88
anaphylactic shock, ix, 101
anastomosis, 33, 37, 38
anatomy, 33, 38, 42, 84
anemia, ix, 41, 49, 101, 110, 111
anesthesiologist, ix, 78
anesthetics, ix, 77, 88, 89, 97, 102, 111
angiogenesis, 24, 85, 87, 93, 94, 98
angiotensin converting enzyme, 65

</td></tr>
</table>

angiotensin receptor blockers, 65
anhydrase, 128
antacids, 130
antibody, 92, 105
anticoagulant, 111
antigen, 11, 13, 14, 104, 105, 106, 114
anti-inflammatory drugs, 96, 97
antireflux barrier, ix, 119
antitumor, 92, 96, 97
antitumor immunity, 92
APC, 82
apoptosis, 3, 7, 14, 22, 66, 85, 87, 94, 96, 97
appetite, 4, 32, 46
Argentina, 154
arrhythmia, 53, 54, 56, 58, 62, 63, 64, 65,
    71, 72, 73, 74
artery, 62, 64, 69, 70, 71, 72, 122
ascorbic acid, 57, 67
aspirate, 152
aspiration, 127, 128, 150
assessment, 46, 137, 149
asthma, 124, 128, 135, 137, 139, 148
asymptomatic, 37, 148
ataxia, 41
atherosclerosis, 19
atria, 56, 57
atrial fibrillation, vii, viii, 53, 54, 55, 56, 59,
    62, 63, 64, 65, 66, 67, 68, 69, 70, 71, 72,
    73, 74, 75
atrophy, 15, 29
automaticity, 57

B

bacteria, 11, 14
bacterium, 104
band slippage, viii, 32, 43, 45
bariatric surgery, vii, viii, 14, 15, 31, 32, 34,
    35, 44, 46, 47, 49, 50, 52
bariatric surgical procedures, viii, 32
barium, 38
bending, 123
beneficial effect, 15, 85
benefits, viii, 53, 95, 108, 111, 132
beta-adrenoceptors, 57

betablockers, viii, 53
bicarbonate, 128
bile, 127, 138, 147, 150, 151
bile acids, 127
bile duct, 147
biliary obstruction, 147, 151
bilirubin, 149
biochemistry, 16
bleeding, viii, 31, 36, 38, 42
blindness, 42
blood, vii, ix, 3, 4, 10, 12, 14, 19, 20, 33, 36,
    56, 72, 77, 84, 91, 101, 102, 103, 104,
    105, 106, 107, 108, 109, 110, 111, 112,
    113, 114, 115, 116, 117, 121, 149
blood circulation, 12, 14
blood flow, 3
blood group, 105
blood pressure, 4, 19, 20, 56
blood supply, 33, 102
blood transfusion, vii, ix, 77, 101, 102, 103,
    105, 106, 108, 109, 110, 111, 112, 113,
    114, 115, 116, 117
blood vessels, 3, 10, 84, 121
BMI, 9, 10, 32, 35, 36, 37, 129
body fat, 18, 19
body weight, 4
bone, 12, 41, 50, 145
bone marrow, 12
bone mass, 41, 50
bones, x, 143
bowel, 6, 8, 40, 49
bowel obstruction, 40, 49
bradycardia, 58, 60, 61
brain, x, 4, 92, 95, 143, 145
brain cancer, 95
breakdown, 80, 81
breast cancer, 85, 87, 88, 89, 95, 96, 97, 98
breast carcinoma, 87
breathing, 129, 140
bronchial tree, 147
bronchitis, 124, 135
bronchoconstriction, 128
bronchospasm, 128
Budd-Chiari syndrome, 147
bypass graft, 69

D

O

P

Q

R

S

T

U

V

[33] Belghiti et al., 1986. Belghiti J, et al: Caustic sclerosing cholangitis: a complication of the surgical treatment of hydatid disease of the liver. *Arch. Surg.* 1986; 121:1162-1165.

[34] Saimot 2001. Saimot AG: Medical treatment of liver hydatidosis. *World J. Surg.* 2001; 25:15-20.

[35] Wen et al., 1994. Wen H, et al: Albendazole chemotherapy for human cystic and alveolar echinococcosis in north-western China. *Trans. R. Soc. Trop. Med. Hyg.* 1994; 88:340-343.

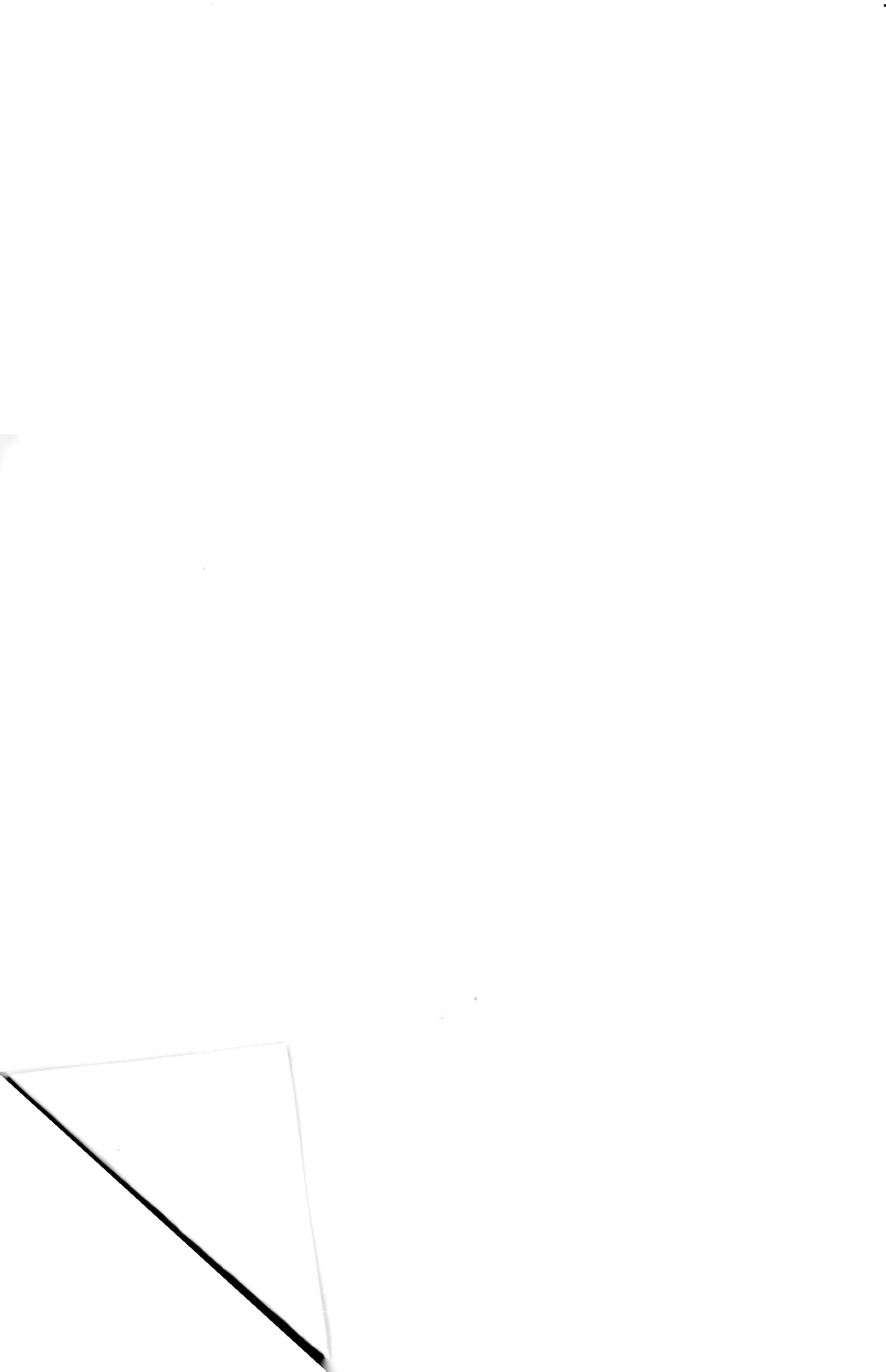

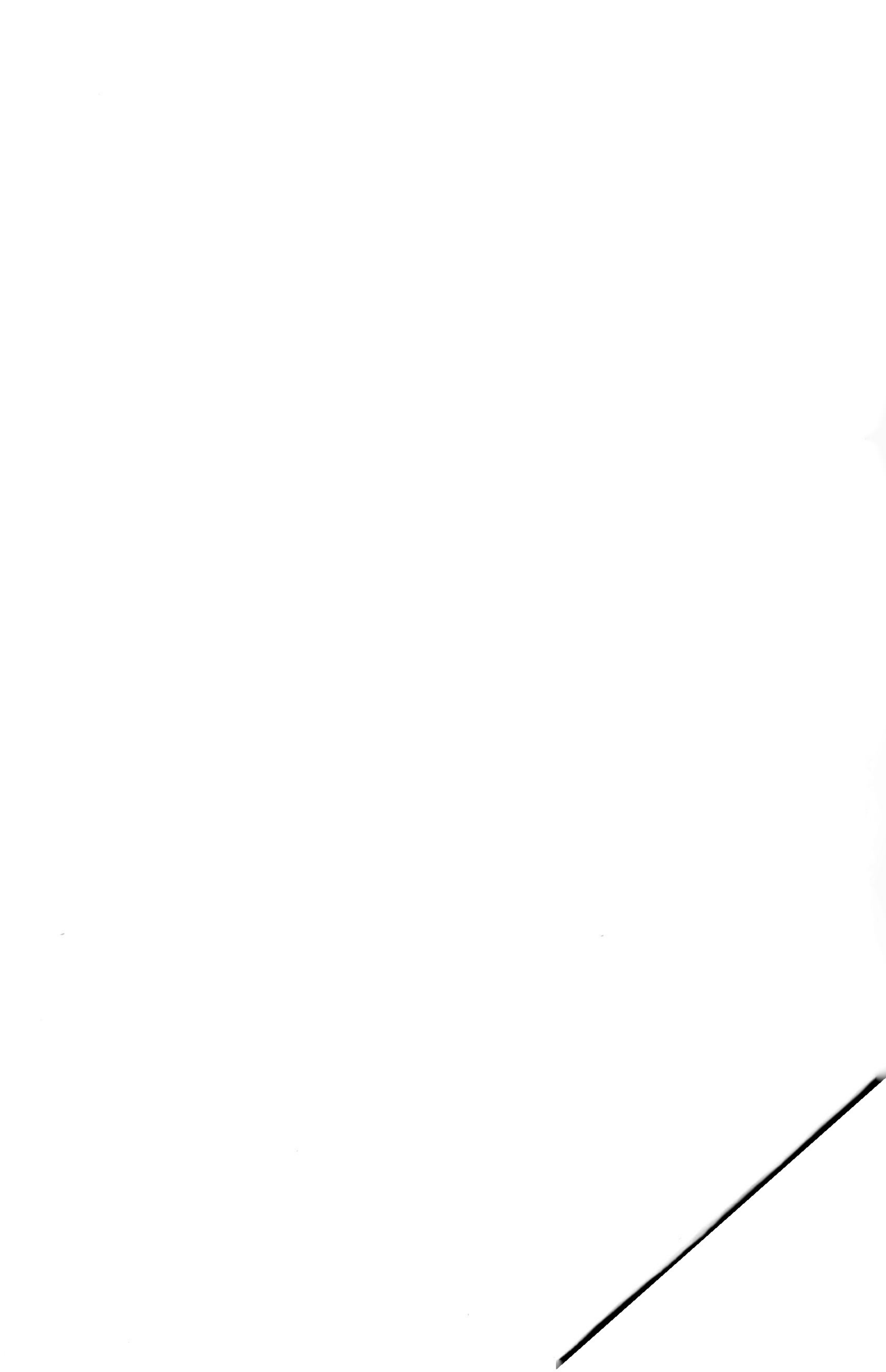